The
Affordable Care
Act

THE
AFFORDABLE CARE ACT

Examining the Facts

Purva H. Rawal, PhD

Foreword by Len Nichols, PhD

Contemporary Debates

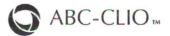

An Imprint of ABC-CLIO, LLC
Santa Barbara, California • Denver, Colorado

Library of Congress Cataloging-in-Publication Data

Names: Rawal, Purva H.
Title: The Affordable Care Act : examining the facts / Purva H. Rawal ;
    foreword by Len Nichols.
Description: Santa Barbara, California : ABC-CLIO, [2016] | Series:
    Contemporary debates | Includes bibliographical references and index.
Identifiers: LCCN 2015036658 | ISBN 9781440834424 (hardback) |
    ISBN 9781440834431 (eISBN)
Subjects: LCSH: Health care reform—United States. | Medical care, Cost of—
    United States. | Health insurance—United States. | BISAC: HEALTH &
    FITNESS / Health Care Issues. | POLITICAL SCIENCE / Government / National.
Classification: LCC RA395.D44 R39 2016 | DDC 368.38/200973—dc23
LC record available at http://lccn.loc.gov/2015036658

ISBN: 978-1-4408-3442-4
EISBN: 978-1-4408-3443-1

20 19 18 17 16   1 2 3 4 5

This book is also available on the World Wide Web as an eBook.
Visit www.abc-clio.com for details.

ABC-CLIO
An Imprint of ABC-CLIO, LLC

ABC-CLIO, LLC
130 Cremona Drive, P.O. Box 1911
Santa Barbara, California 93116–1911

This book is printed on acid-free paper ∞

Manufactured in the United States of America

Contents

How to Use This Book

The Affordable Care Act: Examining the Facts is one of the first volumes in ABC-CLIO's new Contemporary Debates reference series. Each title in this new series, which is intended for use by high school and undergraduate students as well as members of the general public, examines the veracity of controversial claims or beliefs surrounding a major political/cultural issue in the United States. The purpose of the series is to give readers a clear and unbiased understanding of current issues by informing them about falsehoods, half-truths, and misconceptions—and confirming the factual validity of other assertions—that have gained traction in America's political and cultural discourse. Ultimately, this series has been crafted to give readers the tools for a fuller understanding of controversial issues, policies, and laws that occupy center stage in American life and politics.

Each volume in this series identifies 30 to 40 questions swirling about the larger topic under discussion. These questions are examined in individualized entries, which are in turn arranged in broad subject chapters that cover certain aspects of the issue being examined, for example, history of concern about the issue, potential economic or social impact, findings of latest scholarly research.

Each chapter features 4 to 10 individual entries. Each entry begins by stating an important and/or well-known **Question** about the issue being studied—for example, "Did the Affordable Care Act contain provisions for 'death panels'?," "Have scientists established a link between severe weather events and climate change?"

The entry then provides a concise and objective one- or two-paragraph **Answer** to the featured question, followed by a more comprehensive, detailed explanation of **The Facts**. This latter portion of each entry uses quantifiable, evidence-based information from respected sources to fully address each question and provide readers with the information they need to be informed citizens. Importantly, entries will also acknowledge instances in which conflicting data exist or data are incomplete. Finally, each entry concludes with a **Further Reading** section, providing users with information on other important and/or influential resources.

The ultimate purpose of every book in the Contemporary Debates series is to reject "false equivalence," in which demonstrably false beliefs or statements are given the same exposure and credence as the facts; to puncture myths that diminish our understanding of important policies and positions; to provide needed context for misleading statements and claims; and to confirm the factual accuracy of other assertions. In other words, volumes in this series are being crafted to clear the air surrounding some of the most contentious and misunderstood issues of our time—not just add another layer of obfuscation and uncertainty to the debate.

Foreword

Few laws have generated as much intense emotional and ongoing controversy as the Patient Protection and Affordable Care Act (ACA). The law is the culmination of a hundred years of debate, discussion, and attempts at offering near-universal coverage in the United States. Lessons learned from the past, fleeting political majorities, and new policy imperatives to improve quality and reduce ever-rising costs created an opportune policy window in 2009–2010 to pass one of the most expansive—and potentially impactful—pieces of social legislation in our nation's history. However, the very reasons that made health reform necessary and so difficult to pass are also the same reasons that the ACA has divided the nation—both politically and culturally.

In my years as a health economist—working on both the Clinton health reform effort in the 1990s and on the passage and implementation of the ACA, and doing research and speaking about insurance and delivery system reform as well as both legislative efforts all over our large country—I have learned firsthand that few topics are as polarizing as health reform. Over the past several decades, Republicans (mostly) and various sectors of the health care industry have opposed national health reform for fear of government interference and control over health care pricing, decision making, and innovation. They had their specific policy differences, but over time they came to oppose a government strong enough to guarantee health care to all. On the other hand, Democrats (mostly) have chased national health reform because of its potential to make the U.S. health system economically sustainable while serving *all* Americans, not just those with high incomes, those with employer-sponsored health insurance, or those eligible for Medicare or Medicaid. Extending coverage to the uninsured could improve health status and outcomes, improve economic security of families and the government in the long term, reduce health disparities, and even increase productivity among the workforce.

Starting in 2008, when yet another groundswell in support of health reform began to spread among Democrats, the policy and social imperatives to address the problems plaguing U.S. health care system were clear. A record nearly 50 million individuals were uninsured in the wake of the Great Recession, and health care costs accounted for nearly 17 percent of Gross Domestic Product—significantly more than any other nation. At the same time that millions of Americans had no usual source of medical care (or none at all), the U.S. health system also had problems with the quality of care being delivered, especially in managing the chronically ill who are responsible for two-thirds of U.S. annual costs. While both political sides acknowledge and even agree to some extent on the problems facing the U.S. health care system, however, their proposed solutions differ markedly. This division has further exacerbated political tensions between Republicans and Democrats.

The ACA, or "Obamacare," was passed in 2010 after nearly two years of Congressional debate and preparation and a historic Presidential election. More than five years after its passage, however, its legal and policy underpinnings are still called into question, and the law continues to be a political lightning rod. These political divisions, which have manifested themselves in repeated attempts to repeal the law (either entirely or in part) and two prominent Supreme Court rulings, are also reflected in the general public. Public opinion polls have shown a nearly even split in views of the law since 2010.

One of the main reasons for this enduring divide is the lack of bipartisan support for the final version of the ACA. While a limited number of Republicans were key to developing the architecture of the ACA, only two Republicans across both chambers voted in favor of health reform at different points in the legislative process. Most important, no Republican supported its final passage. No other major piece of social legislation in American history has been burdened this way. This stark, party-based divide in support of and opposition to the law planted the seeds for the current biased and politicized public dialogue today.

Supporters of the law—which most notably include the Obama Administration, Congressional Democrats, left-leaning think tanks and policy experts, and progressive leaders of health care organizations in all sectors of the system—point to the significant reduction in the uninsured, the slower growth in health care costs, and the potential for improving population health to justify their position. Opponents of the law, including Congressional Republicans, conservative think tanks and policy experts, and pockets of stakeholder resistance who fear the ACA will reduce their incomes, counter that the ACA is a government takeover of health care. They assert that better policy solutions exist to the problems of rising costs and the uninsured. In fact, on almost all counts, opponents of the law have viewed the ACA as making the U.S. health care system worse in some way—whether by reducing consumer choice in plans, increasing premiums for some, increasing the administrative burden for providers, and ultimately rationing care by focusing on population, not personal, health. While there is truth in both sides' arguments, it is also true that myths, distortions, and inaccurate claims about the ACA have been made by both camps. And the American public has been besieged with these messages ever since the debate over Obamacare began.

The ACA is both a political and cultural issue, and disentangling each side's political rhetoric and cultural values from what the law is intended to do (and its early impacts as implementation is occurring) is difficult—if not next to impossible for the average American. This book is one of the first systematic attempts at examining the credibility of commonly heard and held myths and claims about this landmark law, written by someone who was there when the law was shaped, debated, changed, and passed. Dr. Purva H. Rawal worked for Sen. Kent Conrad of North Dakota, who served on the Finance and Budget Committees, but even more important represented moderate Democratic thinking with a penchant for bipartisan legislation whenever possible. Prior to her service on the Senate Budget Committee, she was the health policy advisor for Sen. Joseph Lieberman of Connecticut—another Senator known nationally for his commitment to bipartisan solutions and independent thinking. Since then, she has worked with a broad range of health care stakeholders on how their organizations may be impacted by—and how they should adapt to—the ACA, including patient advocacy organizations, foundations, insurance companies, pharmaceutical companies, and hospital and health systems. This book is not just for politicos and students but also for the general public. *The Affordable Care Act: Explaining the Facts* tackles 40 myths and beliefs about the law from both sides of the aisle. The book traces the political and historical origins of each claim, and it examines the veracity of each claim using nonpartisan and research-based evidence wherever possible. The book's goal is to provide Americans with a broader understanding of the ACA, fueled by nonpartisan evidence and research, rather than by political rhetoric that often seems impervious to facts or the passage of time.

In the chapters that ensue, a wide range of topics are covered—starting with claims about how the law was passed, its impacts on federal and state budgets, how it limits consumer choice, how it could change coverage for the nearly 150 million Americans who have employer-sponsored insurance, how it may change the health care industry, whether it will improve people's health, and how it is all paid for. While anyone who writes on the ACA has his or her own political leanings, the book truly attempts to give a comprehensive and evenhanded assessment of the wide-ranging myths and claims bombarding the American public. However, the story of the law is still being written—and there are many places where conclusions are difficult to draw. More time is needed before we fully understand if the law can successfully cover more of the uninsured, whether it will succeed in "bending the cost curve" over the long haul and bring health care spending more in line with economic growth, and if it strikes an appropriate balance between government regulation and allowing industry and markets to flourish and innovate.

However, answering these questions requires an informed and engaged American public—and that is unlikely without a deeper understanding of the current debates and controversies over the law. The ACA may or may not have been the "right" answer for our nation's serious health care problems, but it was an answer to the problems of the uninsured, unsustainable costs, and unacceptable quality. This book deserves to play an important part in fostering a dialogue among Americans about what the law set out to do, what is really happening as it is implemented, how it impacts American families, and how all parties can work together to improve U.S. health care system.

Dr. Len Nichols
Director of the Center for Health Policy Research
and Ethics (CHPRE), George Mason University

Introduction

The Affordable Care Act: Explaining the Facts is part of a new series of books aimed at students, policy wonks and experts, and most importantly the general public, on controversial political and cultural issues in America today. Health care reform, and the future sustainability of our health care system—for those in public programs, those with employer-sponsored coverage, or those who continue to be uninsured—is one of the most controversial and complex moral and fiscal public policy problems we face as a nation.

In 2007–2008, when the drumbeat for national health reform first began, the country was falling into the Great Recession, nearly 50 million Americans were uninsured, and health care costs were approaching 16 percent of the Gross Domestic Product (GDP).[1] The long-term impact of health care costs on the federal budget and economy looked even bleaker. At that time, the Congressional Budget Office projected that health care costs could climb to 30 percent of GDP by 2034, accounting for almost $1 of every $3 Americans would spend.[2] No matter what anyone's politics were (or are), the American health care system was spending more money than any other nation, without delivering the same level of value. The social and fiscal imperatives to address both the inadequacies in coverage and unsustainability of costs were pressing.

The Affordable Care Act (ACA) was a legislative response to these public policy problems. The law's passage in 2010 culminated in two years of public deliberations. While some of the deliberations were bipartisan at the start and through much of the law's construction, its passage was partisan, as has been its implementation. At the time of the ACA's passage, few could have imagined the lasting political divisions and partisan public dialogue that would follow the law for years to come, complete with high-profile Supreme Court challenges that upheld key provisions in both 2012 and 2015. The partisan rancor has, unfortunately, resulted in numerous claims and mischaracterizations, and even falsehoods about what the law includes and what its impacts have been and could be. Many of the claims have gained traction and become part of our cultural and political discourse—and this book aims to test the veracity of these claims made by both Democrats and Republicans. Wherever possible, nonpartisan sources and evidence are used to test the veracity of 40 claims about the ACA. The book is divided into eight broad subject chapters, ranging from the passage of the law itself to how it impacts employer-sponsored insurance and labor markets to impacts on consumer choices, the health care industry, and prevention and public health. Some claims end up being true, others are patently false, and for many clear answers have not emerged.

As Americans receive information from more specialized and narrow news sources, it becomes difficult to ascertain or assess politically and ideologically motivated claims and conclusions. It is my hope that this book will serve as a reference for those who are seeking tools for a fuller understanding of health care reform, the issues surrounding it, and the policies that are being implemented. For students, the book can serve as a reference on key ACA issues, as a compendium of health care resources that are respected, and can sharpen their critical thinking and analytic skills as they confront new sets of policy problems to tackle. For policy wonks and experts, much of this may not be new information (and not all may agree with the assessments), but this book may provide some common ground for assessing key parts of the ACA as we all look for answers to improve our health care system. And for the general public, this book may help foster a more complete understanding of the law for both supporters and opponents. For all readers, however, a goal of this book and series is to show the power of assessing the available evidence on public policy issues and using the evidence and data, whenever possible, to arrive at conclusions and solutions.

It has been an honor to write a book that may help cut through some of the partisan noise about the ACA to empower students, policy wonks, and just interested members of the American public to make their own assessments and conclusions about various aspects of the law. There were many individuals who helped move this project along over the past year.

Thanks to my husband, Rahul Tevar, and my two little boys, Shaan and Rami, for encouraging me and being patient while I spent many afternoons and late nights on this project. Thanks also to my mom—Leena Rawal, my siblings, Heeral Valinetz and Kaushal Rawal, extended family, friends and colleagues—whose help and constant check-ins kept me motivated. I would also like to thank a number of individuals who read many parts of this book and gave critical feedback, including Joel Friedman, Madeline Otto Grant, Elizabeth Kelly, Kylie Stengel, and Dr. Michael Stoto. A special thanks to Sabrina Corlette who helped me get all of this started in the first place; Dr. Len Nichols, a respected voice of reason, for writing the foreword; and Dr. John Lyons, who sparked my interest in public policy many years ago. Finally, a sincere thanks to Kevin Hillstrom, a thoughtful editor from whom I have learned a great deal this year, and to the health policy community on both sides of the aisle that I have become a part of and will hopefully continue to learn from, and contribute to, for years to come.

One thing is clear, the story of the ACA is still being written and it will take many years to truly understand the impact, successes, and failures of the law. Hopefully, however, both sides can work together in the coming years to improve on what may be the most impactful piece of social legislation of this generation.

NOTES

1. Centers for Medicare and Medicaid Services. 2014. "National Health Expenditure Projections 2012–2022." Accessed August 21, 2014. http://www.cms.gov/Research-Statistics-Data-and-Systems/Statistics-Trends-and-Reports/NationalHealthExpendData/Downloads/tables.pdf.
2. Congressional Budget Office. 2007. "The Long-term Budget Outlook." Accessed October 13, 2015. https://www.cbo.gov/publication/41650.

1

❖❖❖

Passage and Implementation of the Affordable Care Act

The Affordable Care Act (ACA) was signed into law on March 21, 2010. However, the road to enactment began a few years before in 2008 when Democrats in Congress began to prepare for the possibility of a Democratic presidency. On the Democratic primary campaign trail, health reform had become a key issue among the candidates, suggesting that health reform could take center stage in the nation's capital if one of the candidates were to win. Soon after taking office, President Obama made health reform his top policy priority, stating in his first State of the Union Address in February 2009:

> I suffer no illusions that this will be an easy process. It will be hard. But I also know that nearly a century after Teddy Roosevelt first called for reform, the cost of our health care has weighed down our economy and the conscience of our nation long enough. So let there be no doubt: health care reform cannot wait, it must not wait, and it will not wait another year. (Obama, 2009)

From 2008 through 2010, each chamber of Congress took its own path forward to pass health reform, but in the end any potential for bipartisanship failed and not a single Republican voted for the final bill. The partisan divide has plagued the law's implementation ever since. This chapter examines the myths and claims related to the passage and implementation of the law, including the "deals" cut with industry to allow for the passage of the ACA, the implications of the failed HealthCare.gov rollout in late 2013, and the ongoing regulatory delays the Administration has announced.

Q1. DID PRESIDENT OBAMA AND DEMOCRATS "RAM" THE AFFORDABLE CARE ACT THROUGH CONGRESS AND INTO LAW?

Answer: The ACA did not receive any bipartisan support, and Democratic passage required the use of reconciliation—a budgetary procedure that does not require a filibuster proof majority for the passage of legislation in the Senate. However, the legislative process was not as closed as many Republicans and conservative pundits contend, as the Obama White House and Democratic leaders in the Senate repeatedly signaled willingness to adjust significant elements of the bill in return for GOP support. In addition, Democrats used established, legal Congressional procedures to pass the law—not illegitimate means.

The Facts: Republican members of Congress and conservative pundits alleged that Democrats and the Obama Administration "rammed" the ACA through Congress without public hearings, deliberations, or attempts at bipartisan agreement. From 2008 to 2010, Democrats held the majority in the House of Representatives and a filibuster proof majority in the Senate. While the two houses followed very different paths to drafting and passing their versions of the bill, final passage in Congress was a partisan affair, with no Republicans voting for the final bill in either chamber.

The House set up a Tri-Committee structure to draft the legislation with little Republican input. The Senate process was more bipartisan at the outset, with direct Republican input in the Senate Finance Committee starting with a series of three bipartisan roundtables. In an attempt to garner bipartisan support for health reform legislation, Finance Committee chairman Max Baucus (D-MT) and Ranking Member Chuck Grassley (R-IA) assembled the so-called Gang of Six—three Republican and three Democratic members of the Finance Committee. The group and their staffs met nearly 30 times in the summer of 2009 (Senate Finance Committee, 2010) and crafted the major outlines and provisions of the coverage and financing titles of the ACA (*The New York Times*, 2009). The Health, Education, Labor and Pensions (HELP) Committee conducted a four-week markup of the legislation and accepted over 160 Republican amendments in that time. In addition to the Congressional proceedings, President Obama hosted bipartisan health reform meetings at the White House (beginning with a summit in March 2009), numerous closed-door meetings with members of Congress, and a bipartisan public meeting as late as February 2010 (White House, 2010).

The House of Representatives followed a more partisan process than the Senate, which is unsurprising given the structural differences between the two chambers. The Senate, due to its composition and procedural rules, has historically required greater levels of bipartisanship, whereas the House of Representatives is governed by majority rule due to the rules, precedents, and practices of the chamber (Oleszek, 2011, 28). In the House, three committees—referred to as the Tri-Committee—shared jurisdiction over the various titles of a health reform bill. The Energy and Commerce, Ways and Means, and Education and Labor Committees were all involved in drafting and passage. Speaker Pelosi and her staff closely oversaw this process and held many closed-door meetings with the full committees and relevant subcommittee chairs (Oleszek, 2011, 100). The House released America's Affordable Health Choices Act of 2009 in July and the bill passed the House on November 7, 2009, on a largely party line vote of 220–215. Thirty-nine Democrats voted against the legislation and only one Republican—Rep. Joseph Cao (R-LA) voted for it.

The Senate simultaneously followed its own course. The Finance and the HELP Committees had primary jurisdiction over health reform legislation. The Finance Committee oversaw a process that was bipartisan up until the markup of its bill in September 2009. Beginning in 2008, Chairman Max Baucus (D-MT) outlined the blueprint for the coverage expansion, payment and delivery reforms, and financing of a health reform bill with several hearings, a summit and the release of a white paper, "Call to Action" (Baucus, 2008). Senator Baucus's message at the start of the white paper read,

> It is the duty of the next Congress to reform America's health care system. In 2009, Congress must take up and act on meaningful health reform legislation that achieves coverage for every American while also addressing the underlying problems in our health system. The urgency of this task has become undeniable.
>
> In preparing to act, I led the U.S. Senate Finance Committee in holding nine hearings on health care reform this year and hosted a day-long health summit in June 2008 to explore in greater depth the problems plaguing our health system. I have spent a good deal

of time talking to colleagues on both sides of the aisle and to stakeholders in the health care industry to get their perspectives on the
issues that matter. . . . I have heard from many Americans about the
challenges so many patients and families face in getting access to
affordable health coverage and paying medical bills.

This paper—this Call to Action—represents the next step. (Baucus,
2008)

Following President Obama's election in late 2008, Chairman Baucus
and Ranking Member Grassley (R-IA) plotted out a bipartisan process to
craft a health reform bill. The pair held three roundtables on the main
pillars of the legislation—coverage expansion, payment and delivery
reforms, and financing options. Following each roundtable, the committee publicly released reform options.

However, agreement was difficult to reach across the committee. In
response, Senators Baucus and Grassley convened the "Gang of Six,"
a bipartisan group of Finance Committee members, to reach the outlines of an agreement. In addition to the Chairman and Ranking member, the group included Senators Jeff Bingaman (D-NM), Kent Conrad
(D-ND), Michael Enzi (R-WY), and Olympia Snowe (R-ME). From
June through September 2009, the group and their staffs convened 29
times, for over 60 hours. Their discussion formed the basis for today's
ACA (Senate Finance Committee, 2010). However, the group was
unable to come to an agreement on a bipartisan bill. Consequently,
Democrats brought their own America's Healthy Future Act before
the Committee for markup in late September 2009. Throughout the
markup, the Administration and Democrats heavily courted Senator
Snowe (R-ME) for her vote. They recognized that the media would be
more likely to describe the bill as bipartisan if any Republican vote were
secured—and passage out of Senate Finance Committee was a critical
point in the legislative process. Surprising everyone, Senator Snowe
(R-ME) became the lone Republican vote in the Committee for the
legislation (although she later voted against the final bill when it came
up for a full Senate vote).

That same summer, the Senate HELP Committee initiated a four-week
markup—one of the longest in Congressional history—of another bill
called the Affordable Health Choices Act, which was drafted by senior
members of the Committee over the course of 2009. During the markup,
over 160 Republican amendments were accepted (Health Education Labor
and Pensions Committee, 2009). After the Senate Finance Committee
reported its bill out, the two Committees merged their respective bills

into the Patient Protection and Affordable Care Act, which would eventually go on to become the health reform bill signed into law. The Senate commenced its markup of the legislation on November 30, 2009, and passed it on a party line vote early in the morning on December 24, 2009.

Following passage of the ACA in the Senate, meetings among Democrats in the House, Senate, and White House were convened to merge the bills passed by each chamber. The atmosphere was an exultant one, because it appeared that once they sent a bill to Obama, historic health care legislation that had eluded progressives for decades would finally be a reality.

However, a special election in Democrat-leaning Massachusetts to fill the seat of the recently deceased Senator Ted Kennedy (D-MA) unexpectedly changed the course of events. On January 19, 2010, Republican Scott Brown upset the Democratic candidate in the election to succeed Senator Kennedy, ending the Democrats' filibuster proof majority. With just one stroke, the Democrats' ability to pass health reform was in serious doubt.

The Democrats moved quickly to salvage the legislation. The House agreed to round up the votes to pass the Senate bill and the Senate agreed to pass a second bill with some of the fixes the House would need using reconciliation, a special budget procedure. Reconciliation is intended for Congress to implement fiscal policy—and is usually reserved to reduce spending by reducing entitlement spending and/or cutting or increasing taxes (Oleszek, 2011, 76–77). Its use by the Democrats to pass the ACA, while legal, sparked condemnation from conservatives and is one of the primary reasons that critics of Obamacare allege that Democrats rammed health reform into law.

On March 21, 2010, the House passed the Senate bill and the Health Care and Education Reconciliation Act (HCERA) of 2010, which contained several amendments to the ACA. The Senate immediately took up the HCERA and passed it 56–43, losing the votes of Democratic Senators from conservative states. On March 23, 2010, President Obama signed the ACA into law and the HCERA into law on March 30, 2010. The final votes on the ACA and the HCERA did not garner any Republican support.

The Obama Administration was integrally involved in the drafting and passage of the law in both Houses of Congress. In addition to informal involvement, the President held numerous meetings with members of both sides of the aisle. As late as February 25, 2010 (White House, 2010), he held a bipartisan public meeting at the White House after Senator Brown's (R-MA) election. However, the meeting did not result in any bipartisan compromise, and media reports suggested that at the end of the meeting the President indicated that Democrats would have to move forward without Republican support to pass health reform (National Public Radio, 2010; *The Washington Post*, 2010). In the end, the party line votes on the ACA in both chambers, the use of reconciliation to pass the final bill, the Administration's commitment to passing the legislation even without bipartisan support, and GOP calculations that cries of "foul play" would work to their political advantage all contributed to charges that the bill was "rammed" into law.

FURTHER READING

Baucus, M. 2008. "A Call to Action: Health reform 2009." October 1, 2015. file:///C:/Users/Purva/Downloads/finalwhitepaper1%20(2).pdf

Frakes, V. 2013 "Partisanship and (Un)Compromise: A Study of the Patient Protection and Affordable Care Act." *Harvard Journal on Legislation*, 49: 135–149.

Health Education Labor and Pensions Committee. 2009. "In Historic Vote, HELP Committee Approves the Affordable Health Choices Act." Accessed June 19, 2014. http://www.help.senate.gov/newsroom/press/release/?id=e38929e7-8b99-4df9-9d41-bba123036c94&groups=Chair.

Jacobs, L., and Skocpol, T. 2010. *Health Care Reform and Politics: What Everyone Needs to Know*. New York: OUP.

National Public Radio. 2010. "Bipartisanship Runs Aground at Health Care Summit." Accessed June 19, 2014. http://www.npr.org/templates/story/story.php?storyId=124075675.

The New York Times. 2009. "Health Policy Is Carved Out at Table for 6." Accessed June 19, 2014. http://www.nytimes.com/2009/07/28/us/politics/28baucus.html?_r=0.

Oleszek, W. 2011. *Congressional Procedures and the Policy Process*. Washington, DC: CQ Press.

Senate Finance Committee. 2010. "Health Care Reform from Conception to Final Passage." Accessed June 19, 2014. http://www.finance.senate.gov/issue/?id=32be19bd-491e-4192-812f-f65215c1ba65.

USA Today. 2013. "Obama Wooed Snowe on Health Care—Unsuccessfully." Accessed June 19, 2014. http://www.usatoday.com/story/theoval/2013/04/24/obama-olympia-snowe-health-care-joan-of-arc/2109765/.

The Washington Post. 2009. "Republican Vote Lifts a Health Bill, but Hurdles Remain." Accessed June 19, 2014. http://www.nytimes.com/2009/10/14/health/policy/14health.html.

The Washington Post. 2010. "At Health Care Summit, Obama Tells Republicans He's Eager to Move Ahead." Accessed June 19, 2014. http://www.washingtonpost.com/wp-dyn/content/article/2010/02/25/AR2010022502369.html.

White House. 2010. "A Bipartisan Meeting on Health Reform." Accessed June 19, 2014. http://www.whitehouse.gov/health-care-meeting/bipartisan-meeting.

Q2. DID THE AFFORDABLE CARE ACT INCLUDE "BACKROOM DEALS" WITH INDUSTRY TO ENSURE PASSAGE?

Answer: One of the main reasons experts cite for the failure of the Clinton health reform effort in 1993–1994 was strong opposition from the health care industry. This time, architects of the health reform bill sought to avoid the same outcome and worked to garner industry support—and financing—to the table early on. For the most part, they succeeded in obtaining tacit support from various health industry sectors through an array of compromises—"backroom deals" in Republican parlance—in the provisions of the law.

The Facts: The Obama White House and the Democratic-led Senate Finance Committee worked with the major health care industry sectors to garner their support for a comprehensive health reform bill and to avoid the fate of the 1990s' Clinton health reform effort, which failed at least in part because of strong industry opposition. The basic premise of the negotiations was that insurers, hospitals, pharmaceutical companies, and device manufacturers would benefit from the up to 30 million newly insured lives from health reform; as a result, the industries would partially finance the law. In addition, health industry sectors were convinced that they had to "play ball" with the health reformers, given Obama's support for the cause and the big Democratic majorities that he enjoyed in Congress after his 2008 election. The pharmaceutical and hospital industries publicly announced agreements with the Senate Finance Committee and the Administration in the summer of 2009; however, even before the ACA passed the Senate, media reports with details on the negotiations (especially with the pharmaceutical industry) generated political controversy that continued over the next few years (ABC News, 2009; *Huffington Post*, 2009; *The New York Times*, 2009).

In June 2009, press reports detailed Democratic negotiations with the pharmaceutical industry to convince the latter to support comprehensive health reform and provide $80 billion in concessions to help finance the legislation and improve access to drugs for seniors. In exchange, the industry received guarantees from the Administration that health reform would not include some proposals that the industry was opposed to. As more information surfaced in the media, Congressional Republicans shone a light on the issue. In fact, after Republicans gained control of the House in the 2010 elections, the House Energy and Commerce Committee conducted an investigation into the White House's negotiations with outside interest groups (House Energy and Commerce Committee, 2011). The agreements with industry and negotiations were important in the law's passage; however, any controversy should lie in the nature of the specific deals and agreements themselves—and not that they occurred in the first place.

Legislating has always required deal making between those in government and outside groups, and health care reform was no exception. As Henry Aaron, a longtime health care expert and Brookings Institute fellow, stated,

> Some people who are hawks for going after these groups may not have liked [deals made with the White House], but the Obama administration rather astutely recognized that they could have a greater chance of moving ahead if they weren't being advertised against by a great number of groups that take care of people—and that was worth the price to them. (*The Christian Science Monitor*, 2009)

Beginning in the late spring and into the summer of 2009 as the Senate Finance Committee crafted its bill, the Committee and the Administration negotiated with the pharmaceutical, hospital, insurance, and device industry sectors. The goal was to secure support for a comprehensive health reform bill, which included obtaining industry financing for the coverage expansion that would benefit each of the sectors. Two of the sectors—pharmaceutical companies and hospitals—announced public agreements with the Finance Committee and the Administration in 2009. However, controversy was generated starting soon after when details of the negotiations and tradeoffs surfaced in the media (ABC News, 2009; *Huffington Post*, 2009; *The New York Times*, 2009).

In June 2009, Finance Committee Chairman Max Baucus (D-MT) and the White House announced a deal with the pharmaceutical industry to reduce Medicare prescription drug costs by $80 billion as part of the Democrats' drive to pass comprehensive health reform (Senate Finance Committee, 2009). The agreement included new fees on pharmaceutical manufacturers and policy changes to make drugs more affordable for seniors by addressing the so-called doughnut hole in prescription drug coverage in Medicare Part D. However, press reports surfaced later that summer that in return for the industry's support, the White House had agreed to block any attempts to amend the legislation with certain provisions opposed by "Big Pharma." *The New York Times* reported the story after the industry responded negatively to the House health reform bill, which included policy changes the pharmaceutical industry opposed, such as negotiating drug prices and drug rebates in the Medicare Part D drug program (*The New York Times*, 2009). The industry called on the White House to publicly affirm that it had struck an agreement for $80 billion in cost savings or other contributions to the law and would block any Congressional effort for further concessions (*The New York Times*, 2009).

Similarly, in July 2009, the White House announced a deal with the hospital industry. Hospitals agreed to $155 billion in federal savings to help finance health reform. The reduced federal expenditures came through payment reductions and new payment and delivery reforms aimed at creating a value-based payment system in Medicare (White House, 2009). In exchange, hospitals were allegedly exempted from any further cuts that a proposed oversight board aimed at controlling Medicare spending—the Independent Payment Advisory Board—might make to the Medicare program (*The Christian Science Monitor*, 2009). But just like the pharmaceutical sector, hospitals also had policy priorities for the legislation working its way through Congress. Staffers from Capitol Hill and the White House knew that the insurance industry opposed a public insurance plan option, and that the industry wanted shared responsibility among all stakeholders to ensure the broadest levels of coverage possible (*The Washington Post*, 2009).

However, two sectors did not come to a public agreement with either the White House or the Senate Finance Committee. First, the insurance industry entered into negotiations and agreed to major insurance market reforms, most notably ending coverage denials due to preexisting conditions. In exchange, insurers called for a strong individual mandate requirement to incent young, healthy individuals to enroll in coverage. However, the final individual mandate was weaker than originally envisioned and what the industry felt was necessary to produce stable risk pools of young and healthy, as well as older, sicker individuals. In early October, America's Health Insurance Plans, the primary trade association for insurers, commissioned a report from PriceWaterhouseCoopers on the impact of the Senate Finance Committee's legislation on health insurance premiums (PriceWaterhouseCoopers, 2009). The study projected larger increases in premiums under the health reform bill than without it (PriceWaterhouseCoopers, 2009). The collaboration with insurers was over at this point in the process, and no public agreement was ever made (McDonough, 2011, 79). In addition, the Finance Committee's final bill included $60 billion in fees on insurers to help finance the health reform legislation (Joint Committee on Taxation, 2010).

Second, the device industry never came to an agreement on support and financing for a comprehensive reform bill. The Senate Finance Committee originally included $60 billion in excise taxes on the industry to help finance the legislation; however, the final number included in the bill voted out of the Senate Finance Committee was reduced to $40 billion. The excise tax was further reduced during the negotiations when the merged HELP and Finance bill was on the Senate floor to a 2.3 percent excise tax raising a total of $20 billion in revenue. The final changes were primarily due to pressure from Senators Evan Bayh (D-IN) and Amy Klobuchar (D-MN), who represented states with large medical device manufacturers (Joint Committee on Taxation, 2010; McDonough, 2011, 78). The device tax is still the most contested of the industry fees or payment cuts as the sector continues to push for repeal of the tax.

The ACA's passage was secured at key points in the legislative process because of negotiations and agreements between the Senate Finance Committee, the Administration, and industry sectors. Not only was industry support for comprehensive health reform key to the effort's success, but so was the financing. While the belief that the ACA included "backroom deals" is true, legislating almost always requires those in government to make deals and concessions to obtain the support of key external groups.

FURTHER READING

ABC News. 2009. "What Did the White House Know about the Pharma Deal?" Accessed October 1, 2015. http://blogs.abcnews.com/political punch/2009/08/what-did-the-white-house-know-about-the-phrma-deal.html/.

The Christian Science Monitor. 2009. "Health Care Reform Obama Cut Private Deals with Likely Foes." Accessed October 1, 2015. http://www.csmon itor.com/USA/Politics/2009/1106/healthcare-reform-obama-cut-private-deals-with-likely-foes.

House Energy and Commerce Committee. 2011. "Behind Closed Doors." Accessed June 19, 2014. http://energycommerce.house.gov/behind-closed-doors.

Huffington Post. 2009. "Internal Memo Confirms Big Giveaways in White House Deal with Big Pharma." Accessed June 19, 2014. http://www.huff ingtonpost.com/2009/08/13/internal-memo-confirms-bi_n_258285. html.

Joint Committee on Taxation. (2010). "Estimated Revenue Effects of the Amendment in the Nature of a Substitute to H.R. 4872, The 'Reconciliation Act of 2010,' as Amended, in Combination with the Revenue Effects of H.R. 3590, the 'Patient Protection and Affordable Care Act' ('PPACA'), as Passed by the Senate and Scheduled for Consideration by the House Committee on Rules on March 20, 2010." Accessed June 19, 2014. file:///C:/Users/Purva/Downloads/x-18-10%20(1).pdf.

McDonough, J. 2011. Inside National Health Reform. Berkley and Los Angeles, CA: University of California Press.

The New York Times. 2009. "White House Affirms Deal on Drug Cost." Accessed June 19, 2014. http://www.nytimes.com/2009/08/06/health/ policy/06insure.html?_r=2&hp.

PriceWaterhouseCoopers. 2009. "Potential Impact of Health Reform on the Cost of Private Health Insurance Coverage." Accessed June 19, 2014. https://www.heartland.org/sites/all/modules/custom/heartland_ migration/files/pdfs/26193.pdf.

Senate Finance Committee. 2009. "Baucus, Pharmaceutical Companies Announce Deal to Reduce Prescription Drug Costs for Seniors." Accessed June 19, 2014. http://www.finance.senate.gov/newsroom/ chairman/release/?id=ac2529ba-f5be-44b0-89b8-69a347930277.

The Washington Post. 2009. "Biden Rolls Out Deal with Hospitals to Cut $155B in Costs." Accessed June 19, 2014. http://www.washingtonpost .com/wp-dyn/content/article/2009/07/08/AR2009070802005.html.

White House. 2009. "Background on Today's Health Care Announcement." Accessed June 19, 2014. http://www.whitehouse.gov/the-press-office/background-todays-health-care-announcement.

Q3. DID THE AFFORDABLE CARE ACT INCLUDE MAJOR PROVISIONS AND ELEMENTS THAT HAD PREVIOUSLY RECEIVED SUPPORT FROM REPUBLICANS?

Answer: While Republican opposition to the ACA was unequivocal during and after the law's passage, there are many parts of the law with a history of bipartisan support, as President Obama, Congressional Democrats, and other ACA supporters have repeatedly pointed out. Just prior to the 2012 Presidential election, in fact, President Obama stated that the ACA was a Republican idea, based on the blueprint of the health reform law passed in Massachusetts in 2006 by then Governor (and 2012 Republican Presidential nominee) Mitt Romney (Obama, 2012). Nonpartisan organizations have stated the same—that Congress used the bipartisan health reform law in Massachusetts and lessons learned from the state's effort to inform the national health reform effort, namely its coverage expansion (Henry J. Kaiser Family Foundation, 2012).

Other health care experts have observed that the ACA closely resembles a Senate Republican plan that was unveiled in 1993 as an alternative to President Clinton's proposed health care reforms. That plan, spearheaded by Lincoln Chaffee (R-RI) and Bob Dole (R-KS) and featuring 18 Republican cosponsors, supported individual mandates, reorganized individual and small group markets, and paid for it with Medicare payment cuts and a cap on tax breaks for higher-income Americans covered through employer-sponsored health insurance. All of these elements, though, were condemned by Republicans when they became part of the ACA.

The Facts: The three main goals of the ACA were to:

1. Expand coverage to millions of previously uninsured individuals,
2. Move the U.S. health care system from one that pays for the volume of services delivered to one that pays for value, and
3. Sustainably finance the legislation.

There is significant controversy on major parts of the legislation—especially how coverage has been expanded to previously uninsured or low-income individuals and if the financing of the legislation is appropriate or sustainable in the long term. However, the key components of the coverage expansion are modeled after the bipartisan Massachusetts health reform law, which was passed in 2006 during Governor Romney's (R) tenure (Henry J. Kaiser Family Foundation, 2012). The insurance market reforms, the health insurance exchange, subsidies for lower-income individuals to purchase coverage, and the employer requirements and penalties, among other provisions, became models for the ACA.

The second goal of the ACA, to move to a value-based health care system, has a strong bipartisan history. Title III of the law includes numerous payment and delivery reforms for the Medicare program. The goal of these reforms is to move the historically fragmented payment system that usually pays for volume of services delivered to one that pays for value. Just prior to the health reform markup in the Senate Finance Committee, Ranking

Member Chuck Grassley (R-IA) stated that health reform should include changes to the Medicare program that move the U.S. health care system to one that pays for value over volume (Senator Grassley, 2009). The Medicare payment and delivery reforms in the final law were drafted in the Senate Finance Committee and were not the most controversial parts of the law. However, they may very well have the most lasting effect, with some already showing early signs of slowing-down health care cost growth.

In fact, many of the value-based payment programs authorized in the law had bipartisan support. Toward the end of the Senate Finance Committee's Gang of Six's work together when questions were circling about whether the group would be able to come to a bipartisan compromise, Ranking Member Grassley (R-IA) stated that members of the group had spent hundreds of hours working together to try to craft a health reform bill that would slow down health care inflation and make health insurance more affordable without adding to the deficit (Senator Grassley, 2009). In particular, he called for policy changes that would improve quality and reduce costs in the Medicare program that could then serve as a catalyst for change throughout the health care system—the goal of the reforms included in Title III of the ACA (Senator Grassley, 2009). Following passage of the law, a former Bush Administration official, Dr. Mark McClellan stated that the provider payment reforms in the law were significant and encouraging (*The Washington Post*, 2010). There are numerous payment and delivery reforms in the law, including programs to establish Accountable Care Organizations (ACOs), Hospital Readmissions Reductions Program, Value-based Purchasing for hospitals, penalties for hospital-acquired infections, and pilots for bundled payments, among others. Many of these provisions were crafted in the Gang of Six and have been regarded as trying to accomplish the goals of rewarding value over volume by bipartisan experts.

Exchanges are another central feature of the legislation and are the primary mechanism for expanding private coverage. Exchanges are a regulated marketplace where consumers can go to select and purchase a health insurance plan. While the coverage expansion itself has not received bipartisan support, exchanges are a bipartisan concept. In particular, exchanges were a central feature of the Massachusetts health reform law, and Rep. Paul Ryan (R-WI) has included Medicare exchanges in his annual Congressional budget as a mechanism for reforming the entitlement program (United States House Budget Committee, 2014). Under his plan, seniors could go into Medicare exchanges and choose private health insurance plans. Conservative health policy experts also supported exchanges during the Massachusetts health reform plan, with one writing:

Current law governing health insurance in many states does not work well to control costs or to expand personal access to coverage. Accordingly, state officials who are serious about creating new, consumer-based systems need to create a new legal framework for health insurance. . . . The best option is a health insurance market exchange. A properly designed health insurance exchange would function as a single market for all kinds of health insurance plans. (Moffit, 2006)

While the ACA exchanges have not received bipartisan support, exchanges themselves have been viewed as a mechanism for extending private coverage to individuals on a bipartisan basis.

There are also a number of smaller provisions in the ACA that have historically enjoyed bipartisan support. For instance, community health centers (CHCs) have received broad bipartisan support for decades. CHCs serve more than 23 million patients—most of whom are uninsured, the working poor, or unemployed—and they are a critical safety net provider in 9,000 locations across the United States (National Association of Community Health Centers, 2015). In the ACA, CHCs received $11 billion in new funding to expand their capacity and to build new centers to accommodate the nearly 20 million new patients they expect (National Association of Community Health Centers, 2010).

Another example of a policy change in the ACA with bipartisan support is the expanded use of Medication Therapy Management (MTM), in which pharmacists help manage medications for patients with chronic disease or complex illnesses. MTM programs have been shown to improve quality and reduce overall health care costs (American Society of Health-System Pharmacists, 2014). The MTM section of the ACA was based on legislation with bipartisan support (American Society of Health-System Pharmacists, 2014). Finally, there are a number of other provisions, such as training more primary care physicians, as well as boosting reimbursement for primary care providers that have bipartisan support and were included in the ACA (American College of Physicians, 2011). In short, while there has been nearly unified Republican opposition to the ACA since before its passage, there are a number of major and minor provisions and concepts in the law that have historically enjoyed (and continue to enjoy) bipartisan support.

FURTHER READING

American College of Physicians. 2011. "ACP Urges Congress to Preserve and Improve, Not Repeal, Health Reform Law." Accessed July 9, 2014. http://www.acponline.org/pressroom/health_reform_law.pdf.

American Society of Health-System Pharmacists. 2014. "Fund Medication Therapy Management Programs in the Patient Protection and Affordable Care Act." Accessed July 9, 2014. http://www.ashp.org/DocLibrary/Advocacy/MTM-Programs.aspx.

Henry J. Kaiser Family Foundation. 2012. "Massachusetts Health Care Reform: Six Years Later." Accessed July 25, 2014. http://kaiserfamily foundation.files.wordpress.com/2013/01/8311.pdf.

Moffit, R. 2006. "The Rationale for a State Health Insurance Exchange. The Heritage Foundation." Accessed April 27, 2015. http://www.heritage .org/research/reports/2006/10/the-rationale-for-a-statewide-health-insurance-exchange.

National Association of Community Health Centers. 2010. "Community Health Centers and Health Reform: Summary of Key Health Center Provisions." Accessed May 19, 2015. http://www.nachc.com/client/Summary%20of%20Final%20Health%20Reform%20Package.pdf.

National Association of Community Health Centers. 2015. "About Our Health Centers." Accessed May 19, 2015. http://www.nachc .com/about-our-health-centers.cfm.

President Obama. 2012. "President Obama: Romneycare Was the Model for Obamacare." Accessed July 25, 2014. http://l.barackobama.com/press/release/president-obama-romneycare-was-the-model-for-obamacare/.

Senator Grassley. 2009. "Grassley Comment on Health Care Debate in Advance of President's Address to Congress." Accessed July 3, 2014. http://www.grassley.senate.gov/news/news-releases/grassley-comment-health-care-debate-advance-president%E2%80%99s-address-congress.

United States House Budget Committee. 2014. "The Path to Prosperity: Fiscal Year 2015 Budget Resolution." Accessed July 9, 2014. http://bud get.house.gov/uploadedfiles/fy15_blueprint.pdf.

The Washington Post. 2010. "Mark McClellan on the Affordable Care Act: 'It's an Important Step.'" Accessed July 3, 2014. http://voices.washing tonpost.com/ezraklein/2010/03/mark_mcclellan_on_the_affordab .html.

Q4. DID THE FAILURE OF THE INITIAL AFFORDABLE CARE ACT WEBSITE ROLLOUT THREATEN THE FUTURE OF THE AFFORDABLE CARE ACT ITSELF?

Answer: The problematic launch of HealthCare.gov signaled to many that the ACA itself was a failure. However, the fixes made to the website and robust enrollment indicate that while the problems with the launch were significant, the broader law's basic viability was not threatened, and enrollment quickly recovered to forecasted levels.

The Facts: The cornerstone of the ACA's coverage expansion are the health insurance exchanges, which are regulated marketplaces where consumers can go to shop for health insurance plans that meet the ACA's coverage requirements. They are also the only mechanism through which low- and middle-income individuals and families that qualify for assistance can use premium tax credits to offset the cost of the insurance policies. The Congressional Budget Office projects that 25 million individuals will gain coverage through the exchanges by 2017 (Congressional Budget Office, 2014).

States had the option to either operate their own exchange and website or allow the federal government to do so. In 2014, 15 states and the District of Columbia elected to operate their own exchanges, with varying degrees of success, and the remaining 35 states relied on the federal government to largely operate the exchange in their state, including the online website (Avalere Health, 2013). As a result, the majority of states and Americans were relying on the federal website—HealthCare.gov—to enroll in coverage. However, when the state and federal exchanges launched on October 1, the federal site, HealthCcare.gov, experienced severe technical problems that took weeks to resolve. Millions of individuals tried to access insurance plan information and enroll in coverage, but were unable to do so or required repeated attempts. It took two months for the site to become fully functional. By the Department of Health and Human Services' own estimates, the site did not function approximately 60 percent of the time (Department of Health and Human Services, 2013).

The high-profile and problematic launch of the website led to considerable criticism about the management of the construction of the site, and questions about the long-term success of the ACA. High-profile politicians, such as Texas Governor Rick Perry (R), saw the website rollout as another sign that the law was a "disaster" (Perry, 2013).

In late October, President Obama assembled a team of private-sector experts to turn around the mismanaged effort, led by Jeffrey Zients in a "Tech Surge" (Department of Health and Human Services, 2013). The team oversaw an effort that:

- provided real-time monitoring that could provide instant incident response,
- fixed over 400 software bugs,
- conducted significant hardware updates,

- improved response times from over eight seconds in early October to less than one second on average,
- reduced errors rates from 6 percent to under 1 percent,
- improved system stability to 90 percent, and
- increased the website's capacity to handle traffic (Department of Health and Human Services, 2013).

Then, Secretary Sebelius told Congress that an estimated $677 million was spent on the information technology undergirding HealthCare.gov, which underscored why public and political concerns were mounting in October and November (The Hill, 2013). Congressional Republicans, meanwhile, kept up a drumbeat of criticism, asserting that the disastrous rollout heralded problems with the other reforms in the law (CNN, 2013). In the Senate, the minority staffs of the Finance and Judiciary Committees launched investigations.

The early failure was blamed on hundreds of software problems and poor infrastructure, as well as poor management and oversight over federal contractors and coordination among the various technical teams, lack of testing, and lack of leadership, including the absence of a single decision-making authority (Department of Health and Human

Summary
Achieving a system that runs smoothly for the vast majority of consumers

	Progress Update
Response Time	• Average system response time lower than one second
Error Rate	• Lower error rate, consistently well below 1%
System Stability	• Hardware upgrades and software fixes to support system uptime of 90%+
Rapid Response Team	• 24/7 monitoring and operating center and team in place to ensure optimal system performance and to respond to glitches and unplanned downtimes
Concurrent Users	• Capacity for concurrent user target of 50,000, supporting a minimum 800,000 visits per day

Figure 1.1 Summary of HealthCare.gov Fixes Led by "Tech Surge"
Source: Centers for Medicare and Medicaid Services. 2013. "HealthCare.gov Progress and Performance Report." Accessed November 9, 2015.

Services, 2014; Senate Finance Committee Minority Staff and Senate Judiciary Committee Minority Staff, 2014). The Administration had set a goal of enrolling 7 million individuals through the exchanges by the end of open enrollment on March 31, 2014, but the website troubles had made that goal seem highly unlikely. However, the Obama Administration set a November 30, 2013, deadline to increase functionality for 90 percent of users. After a high-profile and intensive effort to fix the flaws, the Administration met the deadline (*The Washington Post*, 2013).

On May 1, 2014, the Administration released a report announcing that enrollment had exceeded expectations due to a late surge in sign-ups. Approximately 8 million individuals signed up through state and federal exchanges, with 47 percent enrolling in March, the last month of open enrollment (Department of Health and Human Services, 2014).

In mid-April, the assistant secretary for Planning and Evaluation at HHS reported that enrollment had exceeded the Administration's targets (and most public expectations) due to a late surge in applicants. An estimated 8 million individuals enrolled in coverage through the state exchanges and HealthCare.gov (Department of Health and Human Services, 2014). Of those enrollees, 3.8 million—or 47 percent—gained coverage in the last month of open enrollment (Department of Health and Human Services, 2014). One analysis found that exchange enrollment met or exceeded expectations in 22 states (44 percent) (Avalere Health, 2014). This late surge is consistent with enrollment patterns in the Medicare Part D drug benefit program, the Federal Employee Health Benefits Program, and employer-sponsored insurance (Department of Health and Human Services, 2014). The impact of the first year of the ACA's exchanges was a significant drop in the rate of uninsured Americans from 17.9 percent of adults just before the exchanges launched to 13.9 percent after the end of open enrollment, with 8 million individuals gaining coverage (Long et al., 2014). By the end of the second year of open enrollment, the percentage of uninsured Americans had fallen to 11.9 percent according to one poll, which was the lowest on record since the poll began in 2008 (Levy, 2015).

While open enrollment numbers for 2014 were not affected in the end by the rollout, there is a possibility that longer-term impacts could be seen. For instance, there was a possibility that insurance companies would elect to either drop out of or not participate in the new states given the problems with HealthCare.gov the first year. However, this was not borne out either as more insurance companies are seeking to participate in the state and federal exchanges in 2015 and enrollment is also expected to

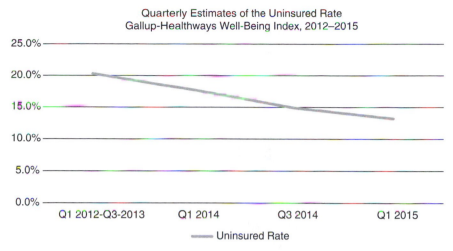

Figure 1.2 Percentage Uninsured in United States by Quarter

Source: Assistant Secretary for Planning and Evaluation. 2015. "Health Insurance Coverage and the Affordable Care Act. Department of Health and Human Services." Accessed July 6, 2015. http://aspe.hhs.gov/health/reports/2015/uninsured_change/ib_uninsured_change.pdf.

grow (*The New York Times*, 2014). In addition, HealthCare.gov should be more functional in 2015 with a new lead contractor. As with many projects, the government has relied on private contractors to build Health-Care.gov. The original primary contractor was CGI, which was awarded a sole source $90 million contract (Congressional Research Service, 2014). However, the contract was not renewed in February 2014 due to the problems with the rollout.

While the website rollout itself was clearly a failure in the first two months after the launch of the exchanges, there was not a discernible long-term impact on enrollment given that the final enrollment numbers for 2014 exceeded the Administration's goals and expert projections. The website launch indicates problems with the underlying technology infrastructure, leadership at HHS, and management of the project; however, it does not signal an overall failure of the ACA itself.

FURTHER READING

Assistant Secretary for Planning and Evaluation. 2015. "Health Insurance Coverage and the Affordable Care Act. Department of Health and Human Services." Accessed July 6, 2015. http://aspe.hhs.gov/health/reports/2015/uninsured_change/ib_uninsured_change.pdf.

Avalere Health. 2013. "Exchange Operational Models for 2014." Accessed July 14, 2014. http://avalere.com/expertise/managed-care/insights/exchange-operational-models-for-2014.

Avalere Health. 2014. "Avalere Analysis: Exchange Enrollment Outpaces Expectations in 22 States." Accessed July 15, 2014. http://avalere.com/expertise/managed-care/insights/avalere-analysis-exchange-enrollment-outpaces-expectations-in-22-state.

Centers for Medicare and Medicaid Services. 2013. "HealthCare.gov Progress and Performance Report." Accessed November 9, 2015.

CNN. 2013. "Contractors Blame Government for Obamacare Website Woes." Accessed July 14, 2014. http://www.cnn.com/2013/10/24/politics/congress-obamacare-website/.

Congressional Budget Office. 2014. "Insurance Coverage Provisions of the Affordable Care Act—CBO's April 2014 Baseline." Accessed July 14, 2014. http://www.cbo.gov/sites/default/files/cbofiles/attachments/43900-2014-04-ACAtables2.pdf.

Congressional Research Service. 2014. "Contractors and Health care.gov: Answers to Frequently Asked Questions." Accessed July 15, 2014. http://fas.org/sgp/crs/misc/R43368.pdf.

Department of Health and Human Services. 2013. "Press Release: Health care.gov Progress and Performance Report." Accessed July 14, 2014. http://www.cms.gov/Newsroom/MediaReleaseDatabase/Press-Releases/2013-Press-Releases-Items/2013-12-01.html.

Department of Health and Human Services, Assistant Secretary for Planning and Evaluation. 2014. "Health Insurance Marketplace: Summary Enrollment Report for the Initial Annual Open Enrollment Period." Accessed July 14, 2014. http://aspe.hhs.gov/health/reports/2014/MarketPlaceEnrollment/Apr2014/ib_2014apr_enrollment.pdf.

The Hill. 2013. "Health care.gov Costs Total $677M." Accessed October 1, 2015. http://thehill.com/policy/healthcare/192761-healthcaregov-costs-at-677m-through-october.

Levy, J. 2015. "In U.S., Uninsured Rate Dips to 11.9 Percent in First Quarter. Gallup." Accessed April 30, 2015. http://www.gallup.com/poll/182348/uninsured-rate-dips-first-quarter.aspx.

Long, S., Kenney, G., Zuckerman, S., Wissoker, D., Shartzer, A., Karpman, M., and Anderson, N.2014. "Number of Uninsured Adults Continues to Fall under the ACA: Down by 8 Million in June 2014." Accessed July 15, 2014. http://hrms.urban.org/quicktakes/Number-of-Uninsured-Adults-Continues-to-Fall.html.

The New York Times. 2014. "Insurers Once on the Fence Plan to Join Health Exchanges in '15." Accessed July 15, 2014. http://www.nytimes

.com/2014/05/26/your-money/health-insurance/insurers-once-on-the-fence-plan-to-join-health-exchanges-in-15.html?_r=0.

Perry, R. 2013. "Rick Perry: You Can't Dress Up the Failures of Obamacare." Accessed July 14, 2014. http://www.dallasnews.com/opinion/latest-columns/20131231-rick-perry-you-cant-dress-up-the-failures-of-obamacare.ece.

Sebelius, K. 2013. "A Technology Surge for HealthCare.gov." Department of Health and Human Services.

Senate Finance Committee Minority Staff and Senate Judiciary Committee Minority Staff. 2014. "Red Flags: How Politics and Poor Management Led to the Meltdown of Helathcare.gov." Accessed July 14, 2014. http://www.hatch.senate.gov/public/_cache/files/e3ff7336-426b-4363-ad41-086ee120a2f1/HealthCare.gov%20REPORT.pdf

The Washington Post. 2013. "Health care.gov Meets Deadline for Fixes, Obama Administration Says." Accessed July 14, 2014. http://www.washingtonpost.com/national/health-science/healthcaregov-meets-deadline-for-fixes-white-house-says/2013/12/01/a3885612-5a13-11e3-ba82-16ed03681809_story.html.

Q5. DO AFFORDABLE CARE ACT IMPLEMENTATION DELAYS PROVE THE LAW IS A FAILURE?

Answer: Implementation delays of an assortment of ACA provisions have stirred significant controversy and motivated opponents to continue to repeal or delay key parts of the law. There are clearly short-term negative impacts of some of the delays on the successful implementation of the ACA, namely for small businesses and insurers that were anticipating a broader risk pool in 2014. However, the long-term impacts of the delays are unlikely to lead to the failure of the law itself, as underscored by robust enrollment in 2014 and the temporary nature of the delays.

The Facts: As October 2014 drew near, the Obama Administration announced a number of delays in implementing various parts of the ACA. The delays affected a number of the coverage-related provisions, including the Small Business Health Options Program (SHOP) exchanges, penalties on large employers, and cancellations of policies that did not meet new ACA coverage requirements. Some of these delays—especially those affecting employers—drew significant criticism from Republicans. Some lawmakers cited the myriad delays as signs that the ACA was a failure (Senate Finance Committee, 2014). House lawmakers called for a full repeal of the law as the delays mounted (House Ways and Means Committee, 2013).

From the passage of the ACA in March 2010 to the launch of the health insurance exchanges in October 2014, HHS issued thousands of pages of regulations and spent hundreds of millions of dollars on implementation efforts. The task at hand was immense—a complete reorganization of the individual insurance market, which served approximately 13 million individuals at any point in time in 2012, and the largest expansion of the Medicaid program since its creation in 1965 (Claxton, Levitt, and Damico, 2014). In addition, the law included numerous changes to the Medicare program, especially new payment and delivery reforms, as well as new taxes and penalties on individuals and small businesses. The ACA made historical changes to the U.S. health care system in a short period of time and the implementation process was not straightforward—or clean. In the short term, implementation has not been as successful as it might have been due to the delays; however, many of the delays have been made in an effort to make implementation of the complex law possible.

Health care spending in the United States accounted for 17.4 percent of Gross Domestic Product in 2012—nearly one out of every six dollars in America's economy (Centers for Medicare and Medicaid Services, 2013). Given the significant role of health care in the country's economy, any changes to the health care system affect numerous stakeholders and often also have unintended consequences. The ACA brought an unprecedented level of change to the U.S. health care system, impacting all parts of the health care industry, individuals, and employers. As the October 1, 2014, launch date for the coverage expansion loomed, the Administration announced numerous delays to individual provisions, with one conservative think tank, the Galen Institute, counting 31 administrative changes to the ACA (Galen Institute, 2015). Some of the prominent delays include:

- a one-year delay to the employer reporting requirements, which delayed the penalties for large employers until 2015 (Mazur, 2013);
- a one-year delay of the online SHOP exchanges, as well as a delay to a key feature of the SHOP exchanges allowing for employee choice in plan selection (Department of Health and Human Services, 2013; Federal Register, 2013);
- allowing policies starting on or before October 1, 2016, slated to be canceled due to noncompliance with new ACA requirements to continue (Centers for Medicare and Medicaid Services, 2014);
- phasing coverage requirements for medium-sized employers between 50 and 100 employees who work more than 30 hours per week (Treasury Department, 2014).

The delays are attributed to a number of reasons, including that there are literally hundreds of requirements on HHS, employers, insurance companies, and exchanges (among other stakeholders) to comply with in a short period of time, making it necessary in some cases to delay provisions that are not well developed. There have also been limited resources for implementation of the ACA due to Congressional opposition to the law, as well as technological limitations given that entirely new reporting and other systems needed to be built (Jost, 2014).

In response to the these delays and mounting criticism of the Administration's handling of the implementation of the ACA, Speaker Boehner (R-OH) announced that the House of Representatives was suing President Obama over his delay of the employer reporting requirements and penalties (Speaker Boehner's Press Office, 2014). The Speaker contended that the delay marked an overreach of Executive Authority. However, legal experts have cited numerous examples of temporary delays in tax reporting and payment requirements by previous Republican and Democratic administrations when deadlines in laws passed by Congress are not workable (Jost, 2014).

The ACA implementation delays have short- and longer-term consequences. In the short term, the delays have made implementation more confusing and arguably less fair for some stakeholders over others. For instance, the delay of the online SHOP exchanges and lack of employee choice of insurance plans until 2015 has meant minimal participation by small businesses. Participation in the federal SHOP is unknown, but even state SHOP exchanges are reporting low take-up rates. California took its SHOP online enrollment site down in February 2014 and at that time reported that only 571 groups were enrolled in the state's SHOP exchange (Covered California, 2014). The SHOP delays have also led to confusion and discouragement among a group that has been waiting for relief from ever-rising health care premiums (Health Affairs, 2014). While the delays themselves are probably not the sole reason that small businesses have not enrolled in SHOP, they are emblematic of a problem with the construct or at least the implementation of this part of the ACA.

Delaying the coverage and reporting requirements (and as a result, the penalties) for employers with 50 or more employees has been much more controversial. The Administration announced the delay because it concluded that the employer penalty could not be enforced until an effective reporting process for the coverage employers are providing to employees was in place (which it was not; Jost, 2014; Treasury Department, 2013). While the delay appeared to be a practical one, House Republicans used it to help pass legislation postponing the individual mandate as well, contending that the employer delay was unfair to individuals who were not receiving a delay in their mandate (Speaker of the House John Boehner, 2013). In the end, employer reporting requirements and penalties went into effect starting 2015, and enrollment in the ACA exchanges in 2014 does not appear to have been affected.

Finally, the delayed cancellation of noncompliant plans was meant to stabilize the individuals' insurance market and mollify consumers who were about to lose their plans on January 1, 2014, many of whom were unable to enroll in HealthCare.gov due to website problems. However, the delay, which was announced after open enrollment began, created confusion among plans and state commissioners of insurance who were concerned about its impacts on enrollment in HealthCare.gov. The short-term impact of the delay was a likely reduction in the number of individuals who enrolled in exchange plans through HealthCare.gov, as they were allowed to remain in their current policies. Whether or not there is a long-term impact on the success of the law itself is unknown, but there are likely some negative impacts from individuals remaining on noncompliant policies and not joining the exchanges on plans who anticipated broader risk pools when they set premiums for those plans in the exchanges. If policy cancellations are allowed to go into effect in 2017, many of those individuals may enroll through HealthCare.gov at that time, softening any long-term impact of the delay.

FURTHER READING

Centers for Medicare and Medicaid Services. 2013. "National Health Expenditure Data: Historical." Accessed July 16, 2014. http://www.cms.gov/Research-Statistics-Data-and-Systems/Statistics-Trends-and-Reports/NationalHealthExpendData/NationalHealthAccountsHistorical.html.

Centers for Medicare and Medicaid Services. 2014. "HHS 2015 Health Policy Standards Fact Sheet." Accessed July 16, 2014. http://www.cms.gov/Newsroom/MediaReleaseDatabase/Fact-sheets/2014-Fact-sheets-items/2014-03-05-2.html.

Claxton, G., Levitt, L., and Damico, A. 2014. "Data Note: How Many People Have Nongroup Health Insurance?" Accessed July 16, 2014. http://kff.org/private-insurance/issue-brief/how-many-people-have-nongroup-health-insurance/.

Covered California. 2014. "Covered California Suspends Small-Business Online Enrollment to Implement Improvements." Accessed July 16, 2014.

http://news.coveredca.com/2014/02/covered-california-suspends-small.html.

Department of Health and Human Services. 2013. "Direct New Path to SHOP Marketplace." Accessed July 16, 2014. http://www.hhs.gov/health care/facts/blog/2013/11/direct-new-path-to-shop-marketplace.html.

Federal Register. 2013. "Patient Protection and Affordable Care Act HHS Notice of Benefit and Payment Parameters for 2014." Accessed July 16, 2014. https://www.federalregister.gov/articles/2013/03/11/2013-04902/patient-protection-and-affordable-care-act-hhs-notice-of-benefit-and-payment-parameters-for-2014#h-141.

Galen Institute. 2015. "50 Changes to Obamacare . . . So Far." Accessed May 19, 2015. http://www.galen.org/newsletters/changes-to-obamacare-so-far/.

Health Affairs. 2014. "Health Policy Brief: Small Business Insurance Exchanges." Accessed July 16, 2014. http://healthaffairs.org/healthpol-icybriefs/brief_pdfs/healthpolicybrief_108.pdf.

House Ways and Means Committee. 2013. "Brady Opening Statement: Hearing on the Delay of the Employer Mandate." Accessed October 1, 2015. http://waysandmeans.house.gov/brady-opening-statement-hearin g-on-the-delay-of-the-employer-mandate/.

Jost, T. 2014. "Obama's ACA Delays—Breaking the Law or Making It Work?" *New England Journal of Medicine*, 370: 1970–1971.

Mazur, M. 2013. "Continuing to Implement the ACA in Careful, Thoughtful Manner." Accessed July 16, 2014. http://www.treasury.gov/connect/blog/pages/continuing-to-implement-the-aca-in-a-careful-thoughtful-manner-.aspx.

The New York Times. 2013. "Option for Small Business Health Plan Delayed." Accessed July 16, 2014. http://www.nytimes.com/2013/04/02/us/pol itics/option-for-small-business-health-plan-delayed.html?ref=robert pear&_r=2&.

Senate Finance Committee. 2014. "Obamacare: Another Day, Another Delay." Accessed July 16, 2014. http://www.finance.senate.gov/news room/ranking/release/?id=b8845bcf-39d1-420c-b40b-dff9d2c0c1fc.

Speaker Boehner's Press Office. 2014. "Boehner: This Is All about Pro-tecting the Constitution." Accessed July 16, 2014. http://www.speaker .gov/press-release/boehner-about-protecting-constitution.

Speaker of the House John Boehner. 2013. "Boehner: Unfair to Delay Obamacare Mandate on Businesses While Leaving Families on the Hook." Accessed July 16, 2014. http://www.speaker.gov/video/boehner-unfair-delay-obamacare-mandate-businesses-while-le aving-families-hook.

Treasury Department. 2014. "Final Regulations Implementing Employer Shared Responsibility under the Affordable Care Act (ACA) for 2015." Accessed July 16, 2014. http://www.treasury.gov/press-center/press-releases/Documents/Fact%20Sheet%20021014.pdf.

Q6. DID CONGRESS INTEND TO PROVIDE SUBSIDIES ONLY TO INDIVIDUALS PURCHASING COVERAGE THROUGH STATE-BASED EXCHANGES—AND NOT THE FEDERAL EXCHANGE?

Answer: No. In 2015 the U.S. Supreme Court ruled in the case of *King v. Burwell* that premium subsidies should be available to all eligible individuals, regardless of whether they purchase coverage in a state- or federally facilitated exchange.

The Facts: In 2015, the Supreme Court heard another major challenge to the ACA with *King v. Burwell*. The legal challenge stemmed from conservative reading and interpretation of the provisions in the law relating to the premium subsidies, and the Internal Revenue Service's (IRS) subsequent implementation.

This challenge had its roots in 2012, when Cato Institute's Michael Cannon, a leading conservative health policy expert, and law professor Jonathan Adler authored an article questioning whether premium subsidies were available to all eligible individuals regardless of whether they purchased coverage through a state or federal exchange (Adler and Cato, 2012). They argued that the ACA was written (and that Congress intended) to offer premium subsidies only to those individuals purchasing coverage through state-based exchanges. They focused in particular on a single phrase in the law's language that stated that premium subsidies be made available to individuals enrolled "through an Exchange established by the State" (Public Law 111-148, 2010). The authors seized on this interpretation to conclude that the IRS had illegally issued regulations to allow all eligible individuals, including those in states with a federally facilitated exchange, to receive premium subsidies (Adler and Cato, 2012).

The Obama Administration asserted that the challenge was without merit. The Administration and ACA defenders in academic and health policy circles argued that Congress always intended for subsidies to be available in any exchange regardless of whether states of the federal government operated the exchange. They described the federal exchange as an obvious "fallback" in the law if states were to choose not to establish their own exchange, and they characterized the challenge as an effort to use a single imprecise phrase in the drafting of the law's language to bring the whole ACA down.

Defenders of Obamacare argued that the phrasing in question did not refer solely to states but that it denoted a "term of art," with Congress intending that it apply to a federally facilitated exchange as well. This matter of Congressional intent was critical. Cannon and Adler alleged that Congress intended to limit access to premium subsidies to individuals in state-based exchanges to compel all states to establish their own exchanges. The Obama Administration, however, argued that the text in question had to be read within the broader context of the entire ACA law (Jost, 2015). It stipulated that Congress would never have limited subsidies to people residing in states with their own exchanges because such an arrangement would create a federal exchange that would inevitably fall into an insurance death spiral. Such a result would cripple one of the ACA's major goals—to create more functional insurance markets.

The Supreme Court's decision to accept the *King v. Burwell* case put much of the ACA, and the coverage expansion in particular, at stake. By 2015, when the Supreme Court agreed to hear this challenge, 34 states relied on the federally facilitated exchange, and only 16 states and the District of Columbia operated state-based exchanges. If the Supreme Court had upheld the challenge to the ACA, nearly 6.4 million individuals would have lost coverage in those states (Henry J. Kaiser Family Foundation, 2015). Given that the loss of subsidies would have resulted in most of these individuals leaving the exchanges altogether, an insurance death spiral was likely for those remaining. The Kaiser Family Foundation analyzed the impact of the loss of the subsidies on the exchange risk pools and estimated that premiums would increase 237 percent if the Court were to side with the plaintiffs (Henry J. Kaiser Family Foundation, 2015).

On June 25, 2015, however, the Supreme Court ruled firmly in favor of the Obama Administration. In a 6–3 decision, the majority held that Congress clearly intended for premium subsidies authorized by the ACA to be available to all eligible individuals, regardless of whether they purchase coverage in a state- or federally facilitated exchange. Chief Justice John Roberts wrote the majority opinion, stating:

The statutory scheme compels the Court to reject petitioners' interpretation because it would destabilize the individual insurance

market in any State with a Federal Exchange, and likely create the
very "death spirals" that Congress designed the Act to avoid. Under
petitioners' reading, the Act would not work in a State with a Federal
Exchange. As they see it, one of the Act's three major reforms—the
tax credits—would not apply. And a second major reform—the coverage requirement—would not apply in a meaningful way, because
so many individuals would be exempt from the requirement without
the tax credits. . . . It is implausible that Congress meant the Act to
operate in this manner. (Supreme Court of the United States, 2015)

The Supreme Court decision ended another period of uncertainty for
individuals, industry, and state and federal governments about the ACA.
Importantly, the decision affirmed the law again with a sizable majority
ruling.

FURTHER READING

Adler, J., and Cato, M. 2012. Taxation without Representation: The Ille-
gal IRS Rule to Expand Tax Credits under the PPACA. *Health Matrix:
Journal of Law-Medicine*, 23, 1: 119–195.
Henry J. Kaiser Family Foundation. 2015. "State-by-State Effects of a Rul-
ing for the Challengers in *King v. Burwell*." Accessed July 14, 2015.
http://kff.org/interactive/king-v-burwell-effects/.
Jost, T. 2015. "*King v. Burwell*: Unpacking the Supreme Court Oral
Arguments." *HealthAffairs Blog*. Accessed July 15, 2015. http://health
affairs.org/blog/2015/03/05/king-v-burwell-unpacking-the-supreme-
court-oral-arguments/.
Public Law 111-148. (2010) The Patient Protection and Affordable
Care Act.
Supreme Court of the United States. 2015. "*King et al. v. Burwell*, Secretary of Health and Human Services, et al." Accessed July 14, 2015.
http://www.supremecourt.gov/opinions/14pdf/14-114_qol1.pdf.

2

❖❖❖

Impact of the Affordable Care Act on Federal and State Budgets

The economic impacts of health reform were—and continue to be—one of the most debated issues related to the law. Democrats and Republicans disagreed vehemently on this issue throughout the debate and passage of the law, and have continued to disagree about its budgetary impact during its implementation. While official Congressional Budget Office (CBO) estimates projected that the Affordable Care Act (ACA) would decrease the deficit—and that repealing the law would increase the deficit—Republican lawmakers charged that the law was having a negative effect on economic growth, amid the slow recovery. Republican Speaker John Boehner drove much of this message in the House, with statements such as,

> Let's stop payment on this check before it can destroy more jobs and put us in an even deeper hole. Then let's work together to put in place reforms that lower costs without destroying jobs or bankrupting this government. (Boehner, 2011)

This chapter focuses on the debate between the two parties on the economic impacts of the ACA on federal and state governments—including its impact on the federal deficit in the near- and long term, the cost of the Medicaid expansion to states, and whether the ACA is actually slowing health care costs. Some answers are emerging as deficits have improved, states have expanded Medicaid and are seeing savings, and health care costs have slowed, but the ACA cannot be solely credited (or faulted) for these changes. The only certainty is that the economic impacts of the law are complex—and are still unfolding.

Q7. DID THE AFFORDABLE CARE ACT INCREASE THE SIZE OF THE FEDERAL DEFICIT?

Answer: Not according to the CBO, the highly respected, nonpartisan agency that produces budget projections. In 2012 the CBO calculated that the combined effect of the spending cuts and tax increases contained in Obamacare would actually reduce the deficit by $109 billion over the following decade (this 2012 forecast was the most recent estimate provided by the CBO as of mid-2015).

The Facts: The claim that the ACA will worsen the nation's fiscal outlook by increasing the federal deficit originated with Republicans and politically affiliated conservative think tanks and thought leaders (The American, 2009; Blahous, 2012; Cato Institute, 2009; Holtz-Eakin and Ramlet, 2010, 1136–1141; Senate Budget Committee, 2010). However, the CBO projected in 2010 that the ACA would reduce the deficit by $124 billion from 2010 to 2019 (Congressional Budget Office, 2010a). The House of Representatives made repeated attempts to repeal the ACA, which required CBO to estimate the impact of repeal on the federal budget. A complete 2012 estimate projected that repeal would increase the deficit by $109 billion from 2013 to 2022 (Congressional Budget Office, 2012). The main reason that CBO projects the ACA will reduce the deficit is that while the coverage expansion via health insurance exchanges and the Medicaid expansion will cost over $1 trillion over 10 years, cuts to the Medicare program and the new revenues raised from taxes to cover ACA expenses will raise even more revenue.

However, some nonpartisan government entities have cautioned that the ACA *could* increase the deficit in the long term (outside of the budget period that CBO evaluated), and these forecasts have been seized on by Republican and conservative critics. CBO, the Centers for Medicare and Medicaid Services Office of the Actuary (OACT), the Government Accountability Office (GAO), and the Medicare Trustees have all pointed out that Obamacare's budgetary impact will change if certain cost containment mechanisms in the ACA do not go into effect or are curtailed (Boards of Trustees of the Federal Hospital Insurance and Federal

Supplementary Medical Insurance Trust Funds, 2010; Congressional Budget Office, 2010a; Government Accountability Office, 2013; Office of the Actuary, 2010). In particular, the ACA includes cuts to Medicare payments, and these government organizations have noted that it could be difficult to sustain the productivity increases in health care that will be required in response to the lower Medicare payment rates. Taken altogether, based on CBO's assessment and current projections, the law is not projected to increase the deficit.

Despite these caveats, the ACA *as signed into law* will not add to the federal deficit according to the CBO, which was founded in 1974 to provide independent and nonpartisan analyses of budget and economic issues to support Congressional policymaking. CBO produces numerous reports and hundreds of cost estimates annually using a variety of sources, including data from government statistical agencies, health care surveys, and input from external experts in their fields including academics, think tanks, government experts, and private-sector employees.

Throughout 2009 and into 2010, CBO worked with the relevant Committees in the House and Senate to produce estimates on the various versions of the health reform bills as they moved through Congress. The agency's final assessment of the ACA, released on March 20, 2010, projected that it would reduce the federal deficit by $124 billion from 2010 to 2019 (Congressional Budget Office, 2010a). At the time, CBO estimated that the coverage expansion would cost $938 billion from 2010 to 2019; however, the cost of the coverage expansion was outweighed by targeted Medicare payment reductions, as well as new taxes and penalties in the legislation on individuals and businesses (Congressional Budget Office, 2010a).

From the start of the health reform debate, there was controversy about the ACA's impact on the federal budget both in the short- and long term. Republicans in Congress and conservative think tanks and thought leaders insisted that the fiscal impact of the legislation would be calamitous. They claimed that CBO calculations were based on unsustainable cuts to Medicare, budget "gimmicks," and inaccurate assumptions on health care spending, and that Obamacare would in fact worsen the federal deficit (The American, 2009; Blahous, 2012; Cato Institute, 2009; Holtz-Eakin and Ramlet, 2010, 1136–1141; Senate Budget Committee, 2010).

Such sentiments became a cornerstone of anti-Obamacare rhetoric. Similarly, once the ACA was signed into law, the GOP framed its calls for repeal as an act of fiscal responsibility. For instance, Speaker John Boehner stated:

> I don't think anyone in this town believes that repealing ObamaCare is going to increase the deficit. . . . We made a commitment to the

American people. We're listening to the American people. They want this bill repealed. We are going to repeal it. . . . It will ruin the best health care system in the world. It will bankrupt our nation, and it will ruin our economy! (Human Events, 2011)

This belief bolstered efforts to repeal the law, or key portions of it. However, in 2012 CBO released an estimate of the budgetary effect of repealing the ACA that directly refuted the Republican claims. It projected that repealing the coverage expansion via Medicaid and the tax credits to support coverage through the exchanges would increase the federal deficit. CBO concluded the following:

Assuming that H.R. 6079 [a bill to repeal the ACA] is enacted near the beginning of fiscal year 2013, CBO and JCT [the U.S. Congress Joint Committee on Taxation] estimate that, on balance, the direct spending and revenue effects of enacting that legislation would cause a net increase in federal budget deficits of $109 billion over the 2013–2022 period. (Congressional Budget Office, 2012)

CBO attributed the deficit increase mostly to Medicare payment reductions and the loss of revenue from new taxes and penalties (primarily affecting industry players) contained in the law.

However, there are legitimate concerns about the impact of the ACA on the federal budget in the long term. Nonpartisan government agencies, including the CBO, have expressed uncertainty about whether or not the ACA will reduce the deficit in the long term. In 2010, CBO stated that while the agency can provide a detailed examination of the impact of the ACA on the federal budget for the next 10 years, it does not have a reliable analytic method for predicting the impacts of the ACA on federal spending over the long term because a number of factors could affect that spending (Congressional Budget Office, 2010b). In fact, in the 2013 Long-Term Budget Outlook, CBO stated that future spending on health care poses a significant source of uncertainty to the federal budget (Congressional Budget Office, 2013).

The Office of the Chief Actuary (OACT) of the Social Security Administration also evaluates the impact of new laws and changes to current law on Medicare and Medicaid programs. In 2010, OACT stated that it did not believe the Medicare payment reductions in the ACA were sustainable in the long term (Office of the Actuary, 2010). In 2013, OACT again reaffirmed that not enough is known about the sustainability of the Medicare payment reductions and the new payment and delivery reforms in the ACA to reliably project the law's impact on the federal budget in the long term.

In 2012, the GAO also issued a report on the long-term impact of the ACA on the federal budget. GAO conducted its analysis in response to a request by Sen. Jeff Sessions (R-AL), the Ranking Member of the Senate Budget Committee (Government Accountability Office, 2013). The GAO examined a number of health spending issues in this report, and concluded that while the long-term budget picture improved following the passage of the ACA, the long-term impact depended on whether the cost containment measures in the law remained intact (Government Accountability Office, 2013). In addition, the GAO concluded that in the near term, the ACA coverage expansion is driving health care spending increases, but over the long term an aging population and technological advances especially will impact federal spending (Government Accountability Office, 2013).

The Medicare Trustees have also called the sustainability of the Medicare payment cuts to health care providers into question. In 2010, the Trustees in their annual report concluded that while the ACA improves Medicare's fiscal picture "substantially," the longer-term projections are uncertain (Boards of Trustees of the Federal Hospital Insurance and Federal Supplementary Medical Insurance Trust Funds, 2010). The Trustees cited a number of points of uncertainty, including not knowing how effective the payment and delivery reforms included in the ACA would be, whether the Patient-Centered Outcomes Research Institute (PCORI) charged with leading comparative effectiveness research across public and private stakeholders will be successful in impacting health care spending, and whether Congress would override the Medicare payment reductions in the ACA if the cuts prove unsustainable (Boards of Trustees of the Federal Hospital Insurance and Federal Supplementary Medical Insurance Trust Funds, 2010). In 2012, the Trustees reiterated this conclusion and stated that the fiscal picture could look more negative than CBO's projections because the Medicare payment cuts would require unprecedented levels of productivity not seen before from the health care sector (Boards of Trustees of the Federal Hospital Insurance and Federal Supplementary Medical Insurance Trust Funds, 2012).

On the other hand, researchers at the Urban Institute, a DC-based nonpartisan think tank, evaluated CBO's estimates and suggested that while CBO may have been somewhat optimistic in its projections that Medicare payment reductions and new revenues from taxes and penalties will outweigh the cost of the coverage expansion, the agency did not significantly overestimate the fiscal impact of the Act (Holahan, 2010). The

Urban Institute concluded that CBO may have actually underestimated the impact of other provisions in the ACA aimed at controlling costs, such as the Medicare payment and delivery reforms, PCORI, taxes on high-cost employer health plans (i.e., the "Cadillac tax"), and competition among health insurance plans within the exchanges (Holahan, 2010).

In the near term, the ACA does not increase the federal deficit, as Congress included cuts to Medicare and new taxes and penalties on individuals and businesses to offset the cost of the coverage expansion. However, concerns that the ACA will worsen the long-term budget situation are likely to remain, given continued uncertainties about the sustainability of the Medicare cuts in the bills, the impact of long-term cost drivers such as technological changes, and the lack of information on the effectiveness of payment and delivery reforms and other cost containment mechanisms in the law. Compounding these uncertainties, CBO's projections beyond the standard 10-year budget window can vary widely given that economic indicators and other factors that affect federal spending cannot be predicted.

FURTHER READING

The American. 2009. "The Baucus Plan's Phony Deficit Reduction." Accessed June 19, 2014. http://www.american.com/archive/2009/october/the-baucus-plans-phony-deficit-reduction.

Blahous, C. 2012. "New Study: Affordable Care Act Worsens Nation's Already Unsustainable Fiscal Path." Accessed June 19, 2014. http://mercatus.org/expert_commentary/new-study-affordable-care-act-worsens-nations-already-unsustainable-fiscal-path.

Boards of Trustees of the Federal Hospital Insurance and Federal Supplementary Medical Insurance Trust Funds. 2010. "The 2010 Annual Report of the Boards of Trustees of the Federal Hospital Insurance and Federal Supplementary Medical Insurance Trust Funds." Accessed June 19, 2014. http://www.cms.gov/Research-Statistics-Data-and-Systems/Statistics-Trends-and-Reports/ReportsTrustFunds/downloads/tr2010.pdf.

Boards of Trustees of the Federal Hospital Insurance and Federal Supplementary Medical Insurance Trust Funds. 2012. "2012 Annual Report of the Boards of Trustees of the Federal Hospital Insurance and Federal Supplementary Medical Insurance Trust Funds." Accessed May 20, 2015. http://www.treasury.gov/resource-center/economic-policy/ss-medicare/Documents/TR_2012_Medicare.pdf.

Boehner, J. 2011. "SOTU Fact: Obamacare Will Increase the Deficit, Repeal Will Save Taxpayers Billions." Accessed April 23, 2015.

http://www.speaker.gov/general/sotu-fact-obamacare-will-increase-deficit-repeal-will-save-taxpayers-billions.

Cato Institute. 2009. "Will Federal Health Legislation Cause the Deficit to Soar?" Accessed June 19, 2014. http://www.cato.org/sites/cato.org/files/pubs/pdf/tbb-58.pdf.

Congressional Budget Office. 2010a. "Letter to the Honorable Nancy Pelosi on H.R. 4872, the Reconciliation Act of 2010. March 20, 2010." Accessed June 19, 2014. https://www.cbo.gov/sites/default/files/cbo files/ftpdocs/113xx/doc11379/amendreconprop.pdf.

Congressional Budget Office. 2010b. "The 2010 Long-Term Budget and Economic Outlook." Accessed June 19, 2014. http://www.cbo.gov/sites/default/files/cbofiles/ftpdocs/115xx/doc11579/06-30-ltbo.pdf.

Congressional Budget Office. 2012. "Letter to the Honorable John Boehner on H.R. 6079, the Repeal of Obamacare Act. July 24, 2012." Accessed June 19, 2014. http://www.cbo.gov/sites/default/files/cbofiles/attachments/43471-hr6079.pdf.

Congressional Budget Office. 2013. "The 2013 Long-Term Budget and Economic Outlook." Accessed June 19, 2014. http://www.cbo.gov/sites/default/files/cbofiles/attachments/44521-LTBO2013_0.pdf.

Cutler, D. 2010. Don't Miss the CBO's Good News: The Affordable Care Act Will Substantially Reduce the Deficit. Center for American Progress.

Government Accountability Office. 2013. "Patient Protection and Affordable Care Act: Effect on the Long-Term Federal Budget Outlook Largely Depends on Whether Cost Containment Sustained." Accessed June 19, 2014. http://www.gao.gov/assets/660/651702.pdf.

Holahan, J. 2010. "Will Health Care Reform Increase the Deficit and National Debt?" Accessed June 19, 2014. http://www.urban.org/uploadedpdf/412182-health-reform-deficit.pdf.

Holtz-Eakin, D., and Ramlet, M. 2010. "Health Care Reform Is Likely to Widen Federal Budget Deficits, Not Reduce Them." *Health Affairs*, 29: 1136–1141.

Human Events. 2011. "Boehner: Obamacare Will Bankrupt Our Nation." Accessed June 19, 2014. http://www.humanevents.com/2011/01/07/boehner-obamacare-will-bankrupt-our-nation/.

Office of the Actuary. 2010. "Projected Medicare Expenditures under an Illustrative Scenario with Alternative Payment Updates to Medicare Providers." Accessed May 20, 2015. http://www.cms.gov/Research-Statistics-Data-and-Systems/Statistics-Trends-and-Reports/ReportsTrustFunds/downloads/2010TRAlternativeScenario.pdf.

Office of the Actuary. 2013. "Projected Medicare Expenditures under Illustrative Scenarios with Alternative Payment Updates to Medicare

Providers." Accessed June 19, 2014. http://www.cms.gov/Research-Statis
    tics-Data-and-Systems/Statistics-Trends-and-Reports/ReportsTrust
    Funds/downloads/2012TRAlternativeScenario.pdf.
Senate Budget Committee. 2010. "Budget Perspective: The Real Deficit
    Effect of the Health Bill." Accessed June 19, 2014. http://rsc.scalise.
    house.gov/uploadedfiles/2010_03_18budgetperspective.pdf.
Van de Water, P., and Horney, J. 2010. Health Reform Will Reduce the
    Deficit: Charges of Budgetary Gimmickry Are Unfounded. Center on
    Budget and Policy Priorities.

Q8. DOES THE PRICE TAG OF THE AFFORDABLE CARE ACT EXCEED $2 TRILLION?

Answer: Opponents of Obamacare have publicized studies and certain CBO statistics to charge that the overall cost of the ACA exceeds $2 trillion. But supporters of the ACA have dismissed these studies and claims as based on selective data—and they assert that cost discussions are meaningless without acknowledging the various measures taken by the architects of the ACA to fully cover the cost of the health coverage expansion.

The debate over how much the coverage expansion in the ACA actually cost was a source of controversy and disagreement from the start of the debate. In fact, there is still significant disagreement over how much the ACA costs as opponents and supporters of the law have differing opinions on its long-term impact on the federal budget.

The Facts: When the ACA was first passed, the CBO projected that the coverage expansion, which would provide coverage to low-income individuals under Medicaid and make premium tax credits available to lower to middle-income individuals and families to purchase coverage through health insurance exchanges, would cost the federal government $938 billion from 2010 to 2019 (Congressional Budget Office, 2010). However, opponents of the law have released figures dating back to 2010, claiming that the ACA would actually cost $2 trillion or more (Boehner et al., 2011; Capretta, 2010; Pethokoukis, 2012).

The CBO's initial projection on the cost of the law is based on a 10-year estimate, which included four years before the Medicaid expansion and exchanges went into effect. As a result, the cost of the coverage expansion in 2010 when the law passed was $938 billion. Each year that CBO updates the cost of the ACA, this number increases because more years of the coverage expansion are taken into account and because of the generally rising costs of medical care. Republican estimates of the cost of the law took later years into account or asserted that the cost of the law is rising because of the flaws in the law itself—not because of the general underlying cost trends in health care. Meanwhile, Democrats have focused not on the cost of the coverage expansion itself, which is significant, but on the fact that the cost is paid for in the law and does not add to the deficit.

The largest costs in the ACA are attributed to expanding coverage to an estimated 25 million uninsured individuals (Congressional Budget Office, 2015). The coverage expansion has two main components: (1) states have the option to expand their Medicaid programs to cover individuals with incomes up to 133 percent of the Federal Poverty Level (FPL), and (2) federal tax credits are available to individuals and families with incomes from 100 to 400 percent of the FPL to purchase coverage through the health insurance exchanges.

The cost of the coverage expansion has been debated heavily since before the ACA's passage. Generally, Democrats and health care experts supportive of Obamacare have used official CBO estimates and highlighted that the coverage expansion does not add to the deficit. The cost of newly insuring 25 million people is offset by Medicare provider payment reductions, and new taxes and penalties on individuals and businesses. Meanwhile, Republicans and health care experts opposed to the ACA have focused solely on the cost of expanding coverage, using both official CBO estimates and other projections.

CBO produces estimates in 10-year budget windows for all legislation. The shifting budget window, coupled with updated economic assumptions and actual enrollment data in the ACA, will result in changing estimates from year to year that take into account these new data. Figure 2.1 illustrates how the cost of the ACA increases over time to account for the coverage expansion being in full effect in a given 10-year budget window, as well as due to the rising cost of health care (much like inflation). However, since 2010 CBO has continued to project that the net costs of the ACA's coverage expansion will not increase the deficit because they will be outweighed by the other provisions in the law that are intended to reduce federal expenditures or increase tax revenues (Congressional Budget Office, 2010, 2011, 2015).

Conservative opponents of the ACA have provided a wide range of grim estimates on the cost of health reform from even before the ACA became law. For instance, one conservative health care expert stated that full ACA implementation costs over 10 years (i.e., with the Medicaid expansion and premium tax credits for coverage through the exchanges

(billions of dollars, by fiscal year)

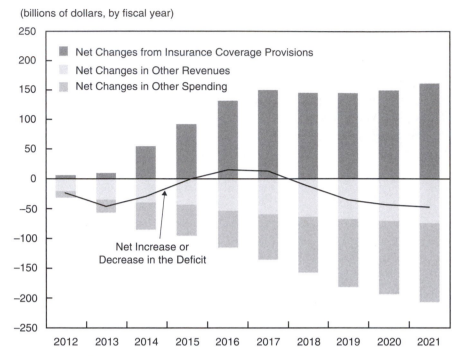

Figure 2.1 Estimated Effects of the Affordable Care Act and Health Pro-visions of the Reconciliation Act on the Federal Budget

with premium tax credits in effect for 10 years) would cost over $2.5 tril-lion (Capretta, 2010). In 2011, Republican House leadership released a report stating that the ACA would cost well over $2 trillion over 10 years of full implementation, stating:

> The government takeover of health care is exacerbating the al-ready dire fiscal challenges our nation faces. If fully implemented, the health care law will cost taxpayers $2.6 trillion, while adding $701 billion to the deficit in its first ten years. By comparison, Pres-ident Obama told a joint session of Congress on September 9, 2009, that he would not sign health care reform that "adds one dime to our deficits—either now or in the future." (Boehner et al., 2011)

There have also been selective presentations of official CBO estimates, with a 2012 analysis pointing out that the gross cost of the coverage expansion could be $2.1 trillion (Pethokoukis, 2012). In this particular case, the $2.1 trillion estimate came from a CBO report on the impact of the ACA on employer-sponsored insurance in which the agency displayed the impacts of range of fiscal and coverage scenarios—and the $2.1 trillion citation was only one of CBO's scenarios.

The primary reason for disagreement on the cost of the ACA is that opponents and supporters of the law are comparing apples and oranges. When the ACA was first passed, the official cost of the coverage expansion was $938 billion from 2010 to 2019, which included six years of Medicaid expansion and premium tax credits for use through the exchanges (Congressional Budget Office, 2010). By March 2015, CBO provided a cost estimate that included 10 full years of the Medicaid expansion and premium tax credits being in effect from 2015 to 2024. In this case, CBO projected that the gross cost of the coverage expansion would be $1.7 trillion, which is the most accurate 10-year cost of the ACA's coverage expansion (Congressional Budget Office, 2015). Opponents of the ACA have cited numbers, stating that the ACA will cost over $2 trillion before CBO's official estimate with 10 years of full implementation was available. As the 10-year budget window CBO uses to estimate the cost of the law moves forward past 2025, the cost will exceed $2 trillion; however, that is not how opponents of the law have explained these estimates and they have not used official CBO estimates in many instances. The higher numbers—and selective use of certain estimates—was part of the opposition's steady campaign to link the ACA to negative economic impacts.

FURTHER READING

Boehner, J., Cantor, E., Camp, D., Kline, J., Ryan, P., and Upton, F. 2011. "Obamacare: A Budget-Busting Job-Killing Health Care Law." Accessed July 25, 2014. http://www.speaker.gov/sites/speaker.house.gov/files/UploadedFiles/ObamaCareReport.pdf.

Capretta, J. 2010. "The President's Health Reform Proposal: More Like $2.5 Trillion." Accessed July 25, 2014. http://www.heritage.org/research/reports/2010/02/the-presidents-health-reform-proposal-more-like-25-trillion.

Congressional Budget Office. 2010. "Letter to the Honorable Nancy Pelosi on H.R. 4872, the Reconciliation Act of 2010. March 20, 2010." Accessed June 19, 2014. https://www.cbo.gov/sites/default/files/cbofiles/ftpdocs/113xx/doc11379/amendreconprop.pdf.

Congressional Budget Office. 2011. "Testimony on Last Year's Major Health Care Legislation." Accessed July 25, 2014. http://www.cbo.gov/publication/25155.

Congressional Budget Office. 2015. "Insurance Coverage Provisions of the Affordable Care Act—CBO's March 2015 Baseline." Accessed March 10, 2015. http://www.cbo.gov/sites/default/files/cbofiles/attachments/43900-2015-03-ACAtables.pdf.

Pethokoukis, J. 2012. "CBO: Obamacare Could Cost $2.1 Trillion through 2022." Accessed May 20, 2015. http://www.aei.org/publication/cbo-obamacare-could-cost-2-1-trillion-through-2022/.

Q9. IS THE AFFORDABLE CARE ACT'S MEDICAID EXPANSION CRAFTED SO THAT INDIVIDUAL STATES BEAR VERY LITTLE OF THE COST?

Answer: Yes, the federal government assumes 100 percent of the costs for the first three years of ACA Medicaid expansion, and 90 percent thereafter.

The Facts: When the ACA became law in 2010, it mandated that all states expand their Medicaid programs to cover individuals or families with incomes up to 133 percent of the FPL. However, when the Supreme Court issued its decision on the constitutionality of parts of the ACA in June 2012, it ruled that states must be given a choice in expanding their Medicaid programs. By mid-2015, 29 states and the District of Columbia elected to undertake the Medicaid expansion, another 4 were considering expansion, and 17 states—all controlled by Republican legislatures and/or governors—had chosen not to expand their programs (Henry J. Kaiser Family Foundation, 2015).

States have opposed (or supported) Medicaid expansion for a number of political and fiscal reasons. Opponents have often cited the cost of the expansion as a reason for not expanding the program. However, supporters of the ACA and governors who have chosen to support expansion (regardless of their political affiliation) have cited minimal costs—and even net savings in some cases—as a reason for expanding their programs. For instance, conservative Arizona Governor Jan Brewer (R) pushed for Medicaid expansion through her state, citing no costs to Arizona and an infusion of $8 billion in federal funding to the state (Brewer, 2013). Nonpartisan analyses of the fiscal impact of Medicaid expansion to states have shown that the costs for those states would be minimal relative to current state spending on the program, and in some cases these studies even project savings to states (Holahan et al., 2012; Dorn et al., 2013). In the end, states that have chosen not to expand their programs have made the decision largely for political reasons and their overall opposition to the ACA.

The Medicaid program is a joint federal–state partnership, with costs for the program split between the two levels of government. Historically, the federal government has assumed an average of 57 percent of Medicaid costs, with the contribution ranging from 50 to 75 percent depending on state per capita incomes (Medicaid.gov, 2014). However, the federal government assumes 100 percent of the costs for the first three years of the ACA Medicaid expansion, which makes individuals up to 133 percent of the FPL eligible for the program. The federal share of the costs of covering the ACA newly eligible beneficiaries then starts to decrease starting in 2017 to 90 percent by 2020. The 90 to 100 percent federal contributions are considerably higher than the average federal contribution for the traditional Medicaid program. As a result, the Obama Administration, Congressional Democrats, and Republican governors that have elected to expand Medicaid cite minimal costs to states.

Despite the significant federal contribution, many states have thus far elected not to expand their Medicaid programs. Republican Governors have led the opposition in many cases. In Texas, Gov. Rick Perry (R) stated:

> Proponents of expansion insist it's a good deal because the federal government will pick up most of the tab, insisting this is "free" money. Texans, however, know there is no such thing as "free" money. We know there's only money that's collected from taxpayers, and money borrowed from other countries like China against the good credit of our children and grandchildren. (Perry, 2013)
>
> Governor Jindal (R-LA) also cited a number of reasons for opposing the expansion, including up to $1.7 billion in costs over 10 years to the state, lack of flexibility in the ACA expansion for states to tailor their programs, and expanding a program whose state funding has doubled in the past 16 years. (Jindal, 2013)

Republican governors and other conservatives have also stated that even if the federal government covers the full cost of new beneficiaries for three years, state costs increase for an already burdened program in the following years. The Heritage Foundation, a conservative think tank, estimated that if all states expanded Medicaid, it would cost them approximately $41 billion over nine years (Senger, 2013). To put this in context, however, the nine-year cost to states is only 6 percent of the total cost of the expansion over that time, making the state investment minimal relative to the federal costs (Congressional Budget Office, 2013).

While projections indicate that the federal government will shoulder the majority of the costs of the expansion, critics are skeptical that state burdens will not increase. Specifically, opponents have raised concerns about whether or not the cost estimates may be higher than what the CBO has projected, if federal funding will be maintained at the levels in the law, and if the federal government will give states flexibility to make changes to their Medicaid programs to meet the unique needs of their populations and state budgets (Payne, 2014).

Governors and legislatures that have thus far rebuffed the ACA's Medicaid expansion deal have also justified their stance by asserting that adding more individuals to their existing Medicaid programs is unwise, given the growing burden of the existing program on their state budgets. Nearly 16 percent of state funds are spent on Medicaid—an expenditure only second to K-12 funding (National Association of State Budget Officers, 2013). As states struggle to balance their budgets, there is understandable concern about adding more beneficiaries—even if the cost is minimal relative to federal costs for a given state.

Supporters of expansion note, however, that state funds are already going to assist those without insurance. The Henry J. Kaiser Family Foundation actually found that overall states are likely to see $10 billion in reduced costs from the Medicaid expansion, primarily due to reductions in uncompensated care (Holahan, Buettgens, Carroll, and Dorn, 2012). In addition, there are a number of other sources of potential savings, including reduced spending on uncompensated care programs for low-income uninsured residents, state-funded high-risk pools, inpatient care for state prisoners, and public health programs, among others (Dorn et al., 2013).

The broader beneficial fiscal effect of expanding Medicaid is a reason that Democrats and Republicans have considered in support of expansion. In Arizona, Gov. Jan Brewer (R) cited the following reasons for supporting Medicaid expansion in her state: (1) no expenses to Arizona, (2) historical public support for maintaining access to Medicaid in the state, (3) keeping state tax dollars in Arizona that would otherwise be spent in other states that are expanding Medicaid, and (4) support for rural and safety net hospitals that provide uncompensated care to low-income uninsured individuals (Brewer, 2013). In her 2013 State of the State Speech, the Governor declared:

By agreeing to expand our Medicaid program just slightly beyond what Arizona voters have twice mandated, we will: Protect rural and safety-net hospitals from being pushed to the brink by their growing costs in caring for the uninsured; Take advantage of the enormous economic benefits—inject 2 Billion dollars into our economy—save and create thousands of jobs; and, Provide health care to hundreds of thousands of low-income Arizonans.

Saying "no" to this plan would not save these federal dollars from being spent or direct them to deficit reduction.

No, Arizona's tax dollars would simply be passed to another state—generating jobs and providing health care for citizens in California, Colorado, Nevada, New Mexico or any other expansion state. (Brewer, 2013)

In this case, Governor Brewer was able to gain agreement from the state legislature, and Arizona expanded its Medicaid program. On the other hand, Florida Governor Rick Scott (R) was unable to convince the state legislature to expand coverage to an estimated 667,000 low-income uninsured residents (Buettgens, Kenney, and Recht, 2014). He cited a number of reasons for expanding Medicaid in Florida, including the fact that Floridians would be contributing to federal taxes that would go to support Medicaid expansion in other states—and that those federal tax funds could be used to assist low-income Floridians instead (Scott, 2013). Governor Brewer's decision to expand Medicaid was controversial, as was Governor Scott's support, but their reasoning suggests that much of the opposition to Medicaid expansion is rooted more in political opposition than in fiscal policy.

In the end, expanding Medicaid has different impacts depending on a state's fiscal situation, its current rate of uninsured, existing uncompensated care programs, and current eligibility for its Medicaid program. However, nonpartisan analyses have concluded that most states are likely to see net savings from ACA Medicaid expansion, that expansion states may also see positive economic effects including increased jobs and revenues, and that hospitals will see increased revenue at a time when Medicare payments are being reduced. One study examined the impacts of Medicaid reform in eight states and calculated $1.8 billion in state savings in just 18 months of the expansion (Bachrach, Boozang, and Glanz, 2015). Finally, while states are concerned about the federal contribution in the long term, Congress has never amended the funding formula to reduce funding to states (Henry J. Kaiser Family Foundation, 2013). Relative to the costs incurred by the federal government for Medicaid expansion, and the potential for enrolled states to realize additional savings from reduced public dependence on other health care programs funded through state dollars, the budgetary benefits of signing up for the ACA's Medicaid expansion are clear.

FURTHER READING

Bachrach, D., Boozang, P., and Glanz, D. 2015. "States Expanding Medicaid See Significant Budget Savings and Revenue Gains." Robert Wood Johnson Foundation and Manatt Health Solutions. Accessed April 20, 2015. http://www.rwjf.org/content/dam/farm/reports/issue_briefs/2015/rwjf419097.

Brewer, J. 2013. "Arizona Governor Jan Brewer's 2013 State of the State Speech." Accessed May 20, 2015. http://www.governing.com/news/state/arizona-brewer-2013-speech.html.

Buettgens, M., Carroll, C., and Dorn, S. 2012. "Cost and Coverage Implications of the ACA Medicaid Expansion: National and State-by-State Analysis." Accessed August 4, 2014. http://kaiserfamilyfoundation.files.wordpress.com/2013/01/8384-slides.pdf.

Buettgens, M., Kenney, G., and Recht, H. 2014. Eligibility for Assistance and Projected Changes in Coverage Under the ACA: Variation Across States. Accessed October 5, 2015. http://www.urban.org/UploadedPDF/413129-Eligibility-for-Assistance-and-Projected-Changes-in-Coverage-Under-the-ACA-Variation-Across-States.pdf.

Congressional Budget Office. 2013. "CBO's May 2013 Estimate of the Effects of the Affordable Care Act on Health Insurance Coverage." Accessed August 4, 2014. http://www.cbo.gov/sites/default/files/cbo files/attachments/43900-2013-05-ACA.pdf.

Dorn, S., Holahan, J., Carroll, C., et al. 2013. "Medicaid Expansion under the ACA: How States Analyze the Fiscal and Economic Trade-Offs." Accessed August 4, 2014. http://www.urban.org/UploadedPDF/412840-Medicaid-Expansion-Under-the-ACA.pdf.

Henry J. Kaiser Family Foundation. 2013. "Quick Take: Key Considerations in Evaluating the ACA Medicaid Expansion for States." Accessed August 4, 2014. http://kff.org/medicaid/fact-sheet/key-considerations-in-evaluating-the-aca-medicaid-expansion-for-states-2/.

Henry J. Kaiser Family Foundation. 2015. "Current Status of State Medicaid Expansion Decisions." Accessed May 20, 2015. http://kff.org/health-reform/slide/current-status-of-the-medicaid-expansion-decision/.

Holahan, J., Buettgens, M., Carroll, C., and Dorn S. 2012. "The Cost and Coverage Implications of the ACA Medicaid Expansion: National and State-by-State Analysis." Accessed August 4, 2014. http://kaiserfamilyfoundation.files.wordpress.com/2013/01/8384.pdf.

Jindal, B. 2013. "Gov. Bobby Jindal: Why I Opposed Medicaid Expansion." Accessed August 4. 2014. http://www.nola.com/opinions/index.ssf/2013/07/gov_bobby_jindal_why_i_opposed.html.

Medicaid.gov. 2014. "Financing and Reimbursement." Accessed July 31, 2014.http://www.medicaid.gov/Medicaid-CHIP-Program-Information/By-Topics/Financing-and-Reimbursement/Financing-and-Reimbursement.html.

National Association of State Budget Officers. 2013. "Summary: NASBO State Expenditure Report." Accessed August 4, 2014. http://www.nasbo.org/sites/default/files/State%20Expenditure%20Report-Summary.pdf.

Payne, A. 2014. "States Begin to Face Overwhelming Obamacare Reality." Accessed August 4, 2014. http://dailysignal.com/2014/05/16/states-begin-to-face-overwhelming-obamacare-reality-medicaid-expansion/.

Perry, R. 2013. "Gov. Perry Takes Firm Stance against Medicaid Expansion." Accessed August 4, 2014. http://www.lrl.state.tx.us/scanned/govdocs/Rick%20Perry/2013/speech040113.pdf.

Scott, R. 2013. "Governor Rick Scott: We Must Protect the Uninsured and Florida Taxpayers with Limited Medicaid Expansion." Accessed August 4, 2014. http://www.flgov.com/wp-content/uploads/2013/02/2-20-13-REMARKSFORDELIVERY.pdf.

Senger, A. 2013. "10 Myths about the Obamacare Medicaid Expansion." Accessed August 4, 2014. http://dailysignal.com/2013/04/24/10-myths-about-the-obamacare-medicaid-expansion/.

Q10. CAN THE REDUCTIONS IN MEDICARE COSTS CONTAINED IN THE AFFORDABLE CARE ACT FINANCE COVERAGE EXPANSION AND EXTEND THE LIFE OF THE PROGRAM?

Answer: Yes, this is one of the main mechanisms by which the health reform law is reducing the deficit. Reductions in Medicare costs partially offset the coverage expansion, but also improve the federal budget picture generally (including the Medicare Trust Fund).

The Facts: When the ACA was signed into law by President Obama in 2010, CBO estimated that provisions in the law would reduce Medicare spending by over $400 billion from 2010 to 2019 (Congressional Budget Office, 2010). The majority of these cuts come from reductions to Medicare provider payments and changes in the way private Medicare Advantage plans are paid. These payment reductions were politically controversial. Opponents of the law charged that the Medicare program was being "raided" to expand coverage to the uninsured. ACA supporters claimed that the Medicare cuts were improving the Medicare Hospital

Insurance (HI) Trust Fund, which at the time only had sufficient funding to remain solvent until 2017 (Foster, 2010). With CBO projecting that the ACA as a whole would reduce the federal deficit, both argued about whether the Medicare payment reductions could be used to offset the cost of the coverage expansion in the law (and help reduce the deficit), while also generally strengthening the Medicare program.

Criticisms of how the Medicare payment changes were being used were leveled both by Republican politicians and by some budget experts. Republican Presidential nominee Gov. Mitt Romney charged that the ACA "robbed Medicare" to finance the coverage expansion (Romney, 2012). Others asserted that the ACA was fiscally irresponsible because the Medicare savings were being used both for new health programs and to strengthen the Medicare Trust Fund (Penny, 2010). A Republican budget expert, Charles Blahous, also released a report in 2012 bolstering the perspective that the ACA could not both reduce the deficit and extend the life of the Medicare HI trust fund (Blahous, 2012).

Defenders of the Medicare cuts, however, pointed out that the CBO had evaluated the fiscal impacts of the ACA on both the federal budget and Medicare HI Trust Fund using long-standing budget accounting conventions. And according to that CBO analysis, the ACA was perfectly capable of having a favorable impact on both the federal deficit and the solvency of the Medicare HI Trust Fund (Congressional Budget Office, 2010).

As the CBO noted, the ACA includes numerous mechanisms for financing the law's Medicaid and private insurance expansion, which the agency estimated would cost $938 billion. The law included over $400 billion in payment reductions to Medicare providers and private plans (Congressional Budget Office, 2010). In addition, the ACA included numerous other changes to federal law and new taxes and fees on individuals and businesses. These changes, combined with the Medicare cuts, more than offset the cost of the coverage expansion and therefore could be viewed as, on balance, producing a reduction in the federal deficit.

However, changes to any law that affect the Medicare program also affect the Medicare HI Trust Fund and the long-term solvency of the program. In this case, the CMS Office of the Actuary (OACT) projected that the Medicare Hospital Insurance Trust Fund would be extended by 12 years—from 2017 to 2029 as a result of the payment reductions in the ACA (CMS Office of the Actuary, 2010).

Critics have argued that the changes to Medicare cannot be used to extend the life of the Medicare program, while also partially offsetting the cost of the coverage expansion and contributing to the deficit reduction resulting from the law. Essentially, they expressed concerns that Democrats and supporters of the ACA were "double-counting" the savings from the changes to Medicare by saying that they both helped finance the coverage expansion and reduced the deficit and also strengthened the Medicare program. The Obama White House, Democrats, and other supporters of the ACA flatly denied the accusation.

While this is a technical issue, it is important because the Medicare program and changes to it are often used for political means by both parties. Basically, the changes to the Medicare program included in the ACA help offset the cost of the coverage expansion and improve the federal budget picture (which includes the Medicare Trust Fund) relative to the ACA not becoming law. The payment reductions and revenue increases from the new taxes are accounted for using a long-standing federal budget accounting mechanism termed "unified budget accounting." CBO uses unified budget accounting to assess the impact of a piece of legislation on federal government finances as a whole, indicating whether it will improve or worsen the deficit. Health economist Dr. Len Nichols examined the criticisms of CBO's approach to examining the fiscal impacts of the ACA and concluded:

> The ACA has many moving parts, and unified budget accounting is the best (and only legal) way to analyze them, as CBO has always done. It is a complex piece of legislation, changing insurance market rules to enable access to all regardless of health status (a fundamentally moral stance), and financing the necessary subsidies with both Medicare savings and modest tax increases (a fiscally responsible stance).
>
> Opponents should just be honest: they oppose using federal power to shift the requisite resources to make our society more fair and to make our health care system more sustainable. That is a legitimate philosophical position with which I strongly disagree. So be it. . . . But what I cannot sanction is the argument that CBO or any other official body is engaged in subterfuge or deceit in analyzing the effects of the provisions of the ACA for what they are: net deficit reducing and our best hope for starting a decades long process of realigning incentives enough to enable all Americans to gain access to the care they need at a collective price we can afford. (Nichols, 2012)

In the case of the ACA, CBO concluded that the law reduces the federal deficit. It also found that the law has a positive effect on the Medicare HI Trust Fund. One way of understanding the dual effects of the

Medicare changes on the overall federal deficit and the Medicare trust funds as part of the budget is to use an analogy from baseball. When a player hits a home run, it is counted in multiple ways—it adds to a team's score for a given game, and it also counts toward that player's batting average (Horney, 2010; Van de Water, 2011). CBO also addressed this issue and explained that the ACA has favorable effects both on the Medicare program and on the federal budget; however, the positive impact on the budget is smaller than the relative impact on the Medicare HI Trust Fund. As a result, there is improvement in both, but the impacts should not be overstated and long-term federal budget issues remain (Congressional Budget Office, 2009). This last point is critical—the ACA does not solve the long-term federal deficit problem and does not solve all of Medicare's financing issues, but does make moderate improvements to the overall fiscal picture and the Medicare program.

Finally, while charges of double-counting were made against the ACA, this same criticism has not been levied when laws making changes to Medicare were enacted in the past. For instance, Social Security legislation in 1983, the Balanced Budget Act of 1997, and the Deficit Reduction Act of 2005 made numerous changes to Medicare. With all of these laws, Medicare savings were accounted for as improving the nation's overall fiscal picture, which included a positive impact on the Medicare Trust Fund (Horney, 2010; Van de Water, 2011). In this case, opponents of the ACA held the law to different accounting standards than previous pieces of legislation that made changes to Medicare and reduced the deficit.

FURTHER READING

Blahous, C. 2012. "The Fiscal Consequences of the Affordable Care Act." Accessed August 21, 2014. http://mercatus.org/sites/default/files/The-Fiscal-Consequences-of-the-Affordable-Care-Act.pdf.

CMS Office of the Actuary. 2010. "Estimated Financial Effects of the 'Patient Protection and Affordable Care Act,' as Amended." Accessed August 21, 2014. http://www.cms.gov/Research-Statistics-Data-and-Systems/Research/ActuarialStudies/downloads/PPACA_2010-04-22.pdf.

Congressional Budget Office, 2009. "Effects of the Patient Protection and Affordable Care Act on the Federal Budget and the Balance in the Hospital Insurance Trust Fund." Accessed August 21, 2014. http://www.cbo.gov/publication/25017.

Congressional Budget Office. 2010. "Letter to the Honorable Nancy Pelosi on H.R. 4872, the Reconciliation Act of 2010. March 20, 2010."

Accessed June 19, 2014. https://www.cbo.gov/sites/default/files/cbofiles/ftpdocs/113xx/doc11379/amendreconprop.pdf.

Foster, R. 2010. "Estimated Financial Effects of the 'Patient Protection and Affordable Care Act,' as Amended." The Office of the Act. Centers for Medicare and Medicaid Services, Office of the Actuary. Accessed May 20, 2015. http://www.cms.gov/Research-Statistics-Data-and-Sys tems/Research/ActuarialStudies/downloads/PPACA_2010-04-22.pdf.

Horney, J. 2010. "Charge That Health Reform's Supporters Are Double-Counting Medicare Savings Is Nonsense." Accessed August 21, 2014. http://www.offthechartsblog.org/charge-that-health-reform% E2%80%99s-supporters-are-double-counting-medicare-savings-is-nonsense/.

Joint Committee on Taxation. 2010. "Estimated Revenue Effects of the Amendment in the Nature of a Substitute to H.R. 4872, The 'Reconciliation Act of 2010,' as Amended, in Combination with the Revenue Effects of H.R. 3590, the 'Patient Protection and Affordable Care Act' ('PPACA'), as Passed by the Senate and Scheduled for Consideration by the House Committee on Rules on March 20, 2010." Accessed June 19, 2014. https://www.jct.gov/publications.html? func=startdown&id=3672.

Nichols, L. 2012. "Is Health Reform Fiscally Responsible?" Accessed August 21, 2014. http://healthaffairs.org/blog/2012/04/20/is-health-reform-fiscally-responsible/.

Penny, T. 2010. "Op-ed: From a Fiscal Standpoint, Alarm about Health Care Reform." Accessed August 8, 2014. http://crfb.org/document/op-ed-fiscal-standpoint-alarm-about-health-care-reform.

Romney, M. 2012. "60 Minutes: Romney, Ryan Answer Critics of Medicare Position." Accessed August 5, 2014. http://www.cbsnews.com/new s/60-minutes-romney-ryan-answer-critics-of-medicare-position/.

Van de Water, P. 2011. "Testimony: Paul Van de Water, Senior Fellow, Before the Committee on the Budget." Accessed August 21, 2014. http://www.cbpp.org/cms/?fa=view&id=3380.

Q11. IS THE AFFORDABLE CARE ACT BENDING THE HEALTH CARE "COST CURVE"?

Answer: Since the ACA was signed into law, the United States has experienced several years of lower-than-usual increases in health care costs. This trend defied the predictions of critics who insisted that Obamacare would trigger a dramatic surge in the cost of health care. Still, strong disagreement exists as to the degree of credit that the ACA should receive for this phenomenon, given the many variables that factor into the overall financial complexion of the nation's health care system, and whether the slower cost growth can be maintained.

The Facts: Health care cost growth has historically grown at a much higher rate than growth of the overall economy. This long-standing imbalance has led to health care spending constituting an ever-greater share of the Gross Domestic Product (GDP)—and requiring a greater share of individual and family incomes. To provide some perspective on the impact of these cost trends on the U.S. economy, health care spending as a percentage of GDP was 5 percent in 1960; it is expected to reach 19.9 percent in 2022 (Centers for Medicare and Medicaid Services, 2014a, 2014b). When compared with other developed nations, the United States spends far more than any of its counterparts. In 2010, per capita spending on medical care in the United States was 1.5 times higher than that in Switzerland, nearly 2 times higher than that in Germany and 2.6 times higher than that in Japan (Henry J. Kaiser Family Foundation, 2010).

In short, the long-term trajectory of U.S. health care spending has long been unsustainable. The CBO has projected that there will be a "substantial imbalance in the federal budget" over the long-term for a number of reasons, including increased health care spending (Congressional Budget Office, 2014). Specifically, CBO projects that government spending on major federal health care programs will double as a percentage of GDP from 7 to 14 percent over the next 25 years if no changes to federal policy are made (Figure 2.2) (Congressional Budget Office, 2014).

In response, the ACA included a number of measures to try to restrain health care cost growth, including Medicare payment and delivery reforms and the creation of an Independent Payment Advisory Board (IPAB). Whether or not the cost containment mechanisms in the law would actually bend the cost curve has been heavily debated. Opponents have generally asserted that the ACA will increase spending for individuals, businesses, and the government (Republican Study Committee, 2010). Supporters tout the mechanisms in the law for controlling costs—and they have been quick to note that in the first years since the law was signed into law, consecutive years of lower than historical cost growth have been observed (White House, 2013).

But while the slower cost growth observed in the years immediately following the ACA's passage is historic, other factors are at work as well. The primary reasons attributed to slowing health care costs are the Great Recession of 2007, passage of the ACA in 2010, and broader health care

Percentage of Gross Domestic Product

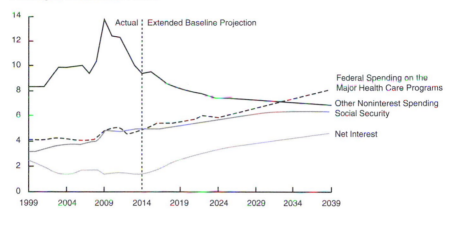

CONGRESSIONAL BUDGET OFFICE JULY 2014

Figure 2.2 Components of Total Spending as Percentage of GDP

Source: http://www.cbo.gov/sites/default/files/45471-Long-TermBudget Outlook_7-29.pdf.

trends. If the slowdown were only due to the Great Recession, then the trend should reverse once the economy is recovering. However, if the ACA precipitated structural changes in the health care system, the slower cost growth trend should be maintained even after the economy has fully recovered.

A nonpartisan analysis examined health care spending trends from 1965 to 2011 to try to determine how much of the current spending slowdown could be attributed to either the Great Recession or the ACA (Henry J. Kaiser Family Foundation, 2013). The Kaiser analysis found that about 75 percent of the decline in health spending growth from 2008 to 2012—the years immediately following the Great Recession—could be attributed to the economic downturn (Henry J. Kaiser Family Foundation, 2013). The analysis also indicated that over the decades, the economy is the largest determinant of health spending; therefore, as the economy recovers health spending, growth also rises again (Henry J. Kaiser Family Foundation, 2013). In addition to the Great Recession, the study cites other possible contributors to the slowdown in health care spending, including greater utilization management from health plans, greater patient cost-sharing in employer and other plans, and delivery system reforms in the ACA (Henry J. Kaiser Family Foundation, 2013).

On the other hand, another study found that the Great Recession accounted for only 37 percent of the slowdown in health care cost growth (Cutler and Sahni, 2013). The researchers found that reductions in private insurance coverage and Medicare cuts accounted for an additional 8 percent of the slowdown, but that 55 percent of the slowdown in spending was unexplained (Cutler and Sahni, 2013). According to this assessment, slower development of new drugs and imaging technologies, higher patient cost-sharing for services and drugs, and increasing provider efficiency all contributed to the trend (Cutler and Sahni, 2013). While not all of these changes are due to the ACA, the changes in provider efficiency likely are.

Other government entities also routinely track health care spending. The CMS Office of the Actuary (OACT) found that in 2013, health care cost growth remained low at 3.6 percent (Sisko et al., 2014). OACT attributed this to continued slow economic growth, impact of federal budget cuts (i.e., sequestration enacted in the Budget Control Act of 2011), slowdown in use of Medicare services, and greater patient cost-sharing with increases in the use of high-deductible health plans (Sisko et al., 2014). However, OACT predicts that from 2014 through 2023 health care cost growth will average 5.7 percent—higher than the years after the Great Recession and the ACA's passage—but lower than the over 7 percent growth seen from 1990 to 2008 (Sisko et al., 2014). The OACT study projects that even after the economy recovers, cost growth will not return to pre-ACA levels, suggesting that other changes are also having an effect. The obvious variables are federal budget cuts, Medicare provider payment reductions, and greater patient cost-sharing; however, longer-term structural changes resulting from the movement to paying for value and not just volume of services delivered—catalyzed and accelerated by the ACA—cannot be ruled out.

The Obama White House concluded that the slower health care cost growth could be attributed at least in part to structural changes in health care—in the way that providers were practicing, for instance—as a result of the incentives and payment reductions in the ACA (White House, 2013). In a press conference after the 2014 midterm elections, for example, Obama stated that

> [d]espite some of the previous predictions, even as we've enrolled more people into the Affordable Care Act and given more people the security of health insurance, health care inflation has gone down every single year since the law passed, so that we now have the lowest increase in health care costs in 50 years, which is saving us about

$180 billion in reduced overall costs to the federal government in the Medicare program. (White House, 2014)

A Center for American Progress (CAP) analysis cited other evidence that the slowdown could be attributed in large measure to the ACA (Volsky, 2013). For instance, CAP reported that premiums for family insurance coverage from 2002 to 2010 (which includes the years immediately after the Great Recession) rose by an average of 8 percent per year, but only by 5.6 percent per year since 2011 (Volsky, 2013). The number of insurers reporting 10 percent or higher rate increases dropped from 75 percent in 2010 to 34 percent in 2012 (Chu and Kronick, 2013). These statistics suggest that the ACA was having a dampening effect on spending above and beyond the Great Recession. However, other prominent health policy experts caution that the jury is still out on the long-term impact of the ACA. They indicate that other broader health care trends, such as consumer-driven health plans with higher deductibles, increasing use of generic drugs, and provider focus on cost containment are also likely factors (Butler, 2013).

Attributing the recent slowdown in health care cost growth to the ACA is difficult, not only because of the Great Recession but also because of other trends in health care (e.g., consumer-driven health plans, slower pharmaceutical innovation). Even proponents of Obamacare acknowledge that more years of data are needed to assess the impact of the law on "bending the cost curve." However, some of the slowdown since 2010 is likely attributable to the payment reductions and value-based payment reforms in the ACA and the pressure they are putting on payers and providers to become more efficient. Whether or not broader health care trends and the changes in the ACA are sufficient to reverse the long-term impacts of health care spending on the federal budget, however, is uncertain.

FURTHER READING

Budget Control Act of 2011. PL. 112-125. Accessed September 20, 2014. http://www.gpo.gov/fdsys/pkg/BILLS-112s365enr/pdf/BILLS-112s365enr.pdf.

Butler, S. 2013. "JAMA Forum: Are Health Costs Really Slowing?" Accessed September 20, 2014. http://newsatjama.jama.com/2013/01/16/jama-forum-are-health-costs-really-slowing/.

Centers for Medicare and Medicaid Services. 2014a. "National Health Expenditure Projections 2012–2022." Accessed August 21, 2014 http://www

.cms.gov/Research-Statistics-Data-and-Systems/Statistics-Trends-and-Reports/NationalHealthExpendData/Downloads/Proj2012.pdf.

Centers for Medicare and Medicaid Services. 2014b. "Table 1. National Health Expenditures; Aggregate and Per Capita Amounts, Annual Percent Change and Percent Distribution: Selected Calendar Years 1960–2012." Accessed August 21, 2014. https://www.cms.gov/Research-Statistics-Data-and-Systems/Statistics-Trends-and-Reports/NationalHealthExpendData/NationalHealthAccountsHistorical.html.

Chu, R., and Kronick, R. 2013. "Health Insurance Premium Increases in the Individual Market." Accessed September 20, 2014. http://healthreformgps.org/wp-content/uploads/rb.pdf.

Congressional Budget Office. 2014. "The 2014 Long-Term Budget Outlook." Accessed August 22, 2014. http://www.cbo.gov/publication/45471.

Cutler, D., and Sahni, N. 2013. "If Slow Rate of Health Care Spending Growth Persists, Projections May Be Off by $770 Billion." *Health Affairs*, 32, 5: 841–850.

Henry J. Kaiser Family Foundation. 2010. "Health Expenditure per Capita." Accessed August 22, 2014. http://kff.org/global-indicator/health-expenditure-per-capita/.

Henry J. Kaiser Family Foundation. 2013. "Assessing the Effects of Economy on the Recent Slowdown in Health Spending." Accessed September 3, 2013. http://kff.org/health-costs/issue-brief/assessing-the-effects-of-the-economy-on-the-recent-slowdown-in-health-spending-2/.

Republican Study Committee. 2010. "Democrats Throw in the Towel on Cost Control." Accessed August 22, 2014. http://rsc.woodall.house.gov/news/documentsingle.aspx?DocumentID=203676.

Sisko, A., Keehan, S., Cuckler, G., Madison, A., Smith, S., Wolfe, C., Stone, D., Lizonitz, J., & Poisal, J. 2014. "National Health Expenditure Projections, 2013–23: Faster Growth Expected with Expanded Coverage and Improving Economy." *Health Affairs*, 33: 10.

Volsky, I. 2013. "The Remarkable Slowdown in Health Care Costs since the Passage of Obamacare." Think Progress. Accessed May 20, 2015. http://thinkprogress.org/health/2013/08/20/2498391/growth-in-health-care-costs-continues-to-decrease-since-passage-of-obamacare/.

White House. 2013. "Trends in Health Care Cost Growth and the Role of the Affordable Care Act." Accessed August 22, 2014. http://www.whitehouse.gov/sites/default/files/docs/healthcostreport_final_noembargo_v2.pdf.

White House. 2014. "Remarks by the President at a Press Conference." Office of the Press Secretary, November 5, 2014. Accessed February 11, 2015. http://www.whitehouse.gov/the-press-office/2014/11/05/remarks-president-press-conference.

Q12. WILL THE AFFORDABLE CARE ACT'S INDEPENDENT PAYMENT ADVISORY BOARD (IPAB) RESULT IN RATIONING IN MEDICARE?

Answer: Concerns that IPAB will lead to rationing care for Medicare beneficiaries are unfounded. IPAB is expressly prohibited from restricting Medicare benefits or eligibility, increasing beneficiary cost-sharing, or raising revenue. The goal in setting up IPAB was to empower a nonpartisan group of health care experts to put policy options in front of Congress to approve (or disapprove) if Medicare spending exceeded targets set in the ACA.

The Facts: The IPAB was included in the ACA to help restrain costs in the Medicare program. IPAB was intended to take some of the decision making over the Medicare program away from Congress and entrust it to a nonpartisan board of health policy experts and stakeholders.

Over the years, the Medicare payment system crafted by Congress had become tied to inefficient and disjointed fee-for-service payment policies. Critics charged that these payment policies were unduly influenced by health care industry constituencies, and that ensuring Medicare's long-term financial sustainability was too often a secondary consideration (Spiro, 2012). A bipartisan group of the country's most prominent health care economists even sent a letter to President Obama in 2009 urging the inclusion in the ACA of a Medicare commission that would make recommendations to Congress to make Medicare more fiscally sustainable and reward health care measures of proven worth in treating health problems (*The New York Times*, 2009).

IPAB eventually became a key cost containment mechanism in the ACA. CBO projected that IPAB alone would reduce the deficit by $15.5 billion from 2010 through 2019 (Congressional Budget Office, 2010). However, its inclusion in the ACA has been controversial, and its implementation has stalled as a result.

Supporters of IPAB describe it as a "fail-safe" that ensures Medicare spending growth will be moderated without requiring Congressional action. One of the key architects of IPAB, former Director of the Office of Management and Budget Peter Orszag, stated that the board reflected the necessity of creating a new process for responding to a changing Medicare payment system that was not just fee for service or volume based (Orszag, 2013). IPAB would provide a new way of controlling Medicare costs—taking into account new data and experience—which is a more dynamic and predictable process than waiting for Congress to act in response to mounting costs and outdated payment systems in many cases (Orszag, 2013). The main Congressional proponent and architect of IPAB, Sen. Jay Rockefeller (D-WV), championed its inclusion in the ACA, stating that the new Board would take "politics and lobbyists out of the business of deciding Medicare payment rates" (Rockefeller, 2010).

IPAB critics, however, charge that the care Medicare beneficiaries receive will be controlled by this bureaucratic board and could lead to rationing of medical care. A prominent conservative think tank stated that IPAB "will have effectively unfettered power to impose taxes and ration care for all Americans" (Cohen and Cannon, 2012). The Ranking Member of the Senate Finance Committee, Sen. Orrin Hatch (R-UT), made a similar charge, stating that the IPAB members would essentially be unelected bureaucrats who could make cuts to Medicare without any transparency or accountability (Hatch, 2012). Some Democrats signaled opposition to IPAB as well. Former Vermont Governor and Presidential candidate Howard Dean (D) expressed concern that the Board would be unable to control costs because he viewed it essentially as a rate-setting entity (Dean, 2013).

The health care industry has expressed widespread opposition to IPAB as well. Given the constraints on how IPAB can reduce expenditures, its primary recourse to keep spending in line with set targets is to reduce Medicare payments. Such reductions would, of course, negatively impact the financial bottom lines of hospitals, physicians, medical device manufacturers, and other industry sectors.

However, some of the criticism directed at the IPAB went beyond what the Board is legally permitted to do. Many Republicans charged that the new entity was a bureaucracy that would control the care that Medicare beneficiaries receive—and even ration care to control costs. Representative Paul Ryan (R-WI), who was also the GOP's Vice Presidential candidate in 2012, stated that IPAB reductions to Medicare provider payments would inevitably lead to rationing (Ryan, 2012). During a 2012 Vice Presidential debate, Rep. Ryan made strong claims that IPAB would directly change the care seniors received, stating:

> And then they put this new Obamacare board in charge of cutting Medicare each and every year in ways that will lead to denied care for current seniors. This board, by the way, it's 15 people, the president's supposed to appoint them next year. And not one of them even has to have medical training. (Ryan, 2012)

Ryan's assertion was that if Medicare payment rates became too low as a result of IPAB, health care providers would no longer treat Medicare beneficiaries—leading to limited access or de facto rationing. Right-leaning think tanks have made similar claims. For instance, there have been claims that IPAB would force widespread payment reductions and give CMS more authority to choose which drugs, devices, and services it will cover (Gottlieb, 2011).

There has also been a strong movement in Congress to repeal IPAB. While mostly garnering Republican support, some Democrats also supported repeal, as do large parts of the health care industry and some patient groups. In 2012, the Republican-led House passed bipartisan legislation to repeal IPAB (Protecting Access to Health Care Act, 2012). Republican Senators have also introduced legislation to repeal IPAB in the Senate, with limited Democratic support, but the measure has never been considered or approved in the Senate (Protecting Seniors' Access to Medicare Act of 2013, 2013).

While IPAB has stirred considerable controversy, the Board has no members and has not had to take any action against rising Medicare costs to date. First, low spending growth in Medicare is keeping spending below targets set in the ACA; therefore, recommendations to reduce spending are not required. Second, the ACA requires members of both parties to nominate appointees to IPAB to ensure a bipartisan (or nonpartisan) makeup. However, the controversy surrounding IPAB from industry, patient groups, and bipartisan members of Congress has stalled any nominations.

Although IPAB could be considered a blunt instrument for keeping Medicare costs in line with targets, Congress has an opportunity to approve recommendations IPAB makes (or pass legislation to keep spending below targets avoiding the need for IPAB to act). The ACA requires that IPAB recommendations go to Congress for consideration under special "fast-track" procedures. At this point, Congress can formally approve the recommendations or take other steps to rein in Medicare costs. If Congress does not act within a set time frame, IPAB's recommendations automatically go into effect. Thus, the criticisms levied against IPAB do not adequately acknowledge that the Board is empowered only when Congress fails to act in order to ensure Medicare's sustainability in the long run. Finally, CBO projected that IPAB would save $15.5 billion from 2010 to 2019—less than 4 percent of the total Medicare savings in the ACA (Henry J. Kaiser Family Foundation, 2011). Some observers speculate that the mere existence of IPAB may be keeping pressure on payer and providers to deliver care efficiently, thereby preventing the need for across-the-board payment reductions or other actions to reduce spending. While the threat of IPAB—even without its official establishment—may be having spillover effects on health spending, there is no evidence that IPAB would lead to rationing services for Medicare beneficiaries.

FURTHER READING

Centers for Medicare and Medicaid, Office of the Actuary. 2014. Letter to Administrator Tavenner. Accessed September 27, 2014. http://www .cms.gov/Research-Statistics-Data-and-Systems/Research/Actuarial Studies/Downloads/IPAB-2014-07-28.pdf.

Cohen, D., and Cannon, M. 2012. "The Independent Payment Advisory Board: PPACA's Anti-constitutional and Authoritarian Super-Legislature." Accessed September 21, 2014. http://www.cato.org/sites/ cato.org/files/pubs/pdf/PA700.pdf.

Congressional Budget Office. 2010. "Letter to the Honorable Nancy Pelosi on H.R. 4872, the Reconciliation Act of 2010. March 20, 2010." Accessed June 19, 2014. https://www.cbo.gov/sites/default/files/cbo files/ftpdocs/113xx/doc11379/amendreconprop.pdf.

Dean, H. 2013. "The Affordable Care Act's Rate-Setting Won't Work: Experience Tells Me the Independent Payment Advisory Board Will Fail." Accessed September 21, 2014. http://online.wsj.com/news/articles/ SB10001424127887324110404578628542498014414.

Gottlieb, S. 2011. "IPAB: The Controversial Consequences for Medicare and Seniors." Accessed September 27, 2014. http://www.aei.org/ publication/ipab-the-controversial-consequences-for-medicare-and-seniors/.

Hatch, O. 2012. "President's Health Law Two Years Later: Raiding Medicare and the Specter of IPAB." Accessed September 21, 2014. http:// www.finance.senate.gov/newsroom/ranking/release/?id=646db6f2-426 e-489d-bd7f-043d02cffd51.

Henry J. Kaiser Family Foundation. 2011. "The Independent Payment Advisory Board: A New Approach to Controlling Medicare Spending." Accessed September 27, 2014. http://kaiserfamilyfoundation.files .wordpress.com/2013/01/8150.pdf.

The New York Times. 2009. "Economists' Letter to Obama on Health Care Reform." Accessed September 29, 2014. http://economix.blogs .nytimes.com/2009/11/17/economists-letter-to-obama-on-health-care-reform/?_php=true&_type=blogs&_r=0.

Orszag, P. 2013. "Critics Are Wrong about the Medicare Payment Board." Accessed September 21, 2014. http://www.bloombergview.com/articles/ 2013-07-30/critics-are-wrong-about-the-medicare-payment-board.

Protecting Access to Health care Act. 2012. Accessed September 27, 2014. https://www.congress.gov/bill/112th-congress/house-bill/5/cosponsors? q=%7B%22search%22%3A%5B%22H.R.+5%22%5D%7D.

Protecting Seniors' Access to Medicare Act of 2013. 2013. Accessed September 27, 2014. https://www.congress.gov/bill/113th-congress/senate-bill/351/cosponsors?q=%7B%22search%22%3A%5B%22S351%22%5D%7D.

Rockefeller, J. 2010. "Rockefeller Hails Passage of Landmark Senate Health Care Bill." Accessed September 21, 2014. http://www.rockefeller.senate.gov/public/index.cfm/2009/12/post-3df51328-bcae-458f-b2c3-b736dddaf353.

Ryan, P. 2012. "October 11, 2012 Debate Transcript." Accessed September 27, 2014. http://www.debates.org/index.php?page=october-11-2012-the-biden-romney-vice-presidential-debate.

Spiro, T. 2012. "The Independent Payment Advisory Board: Protecting Medicare Beneficiaries and Taxpayers from Special Interests." Accessed September 29, 2014. http://www.americanprogress.org/issues/healthcare/report/2012/03/05/11269/the-independent-payment-advisory-board/.

3

❖

Consumer Choices and the Affordable Care Act

Americans generally place a premium on choice in health care. They value having choices among health insurance plans, in the physicians and hospitals they visit, and in the benefits they receive. Unsurprisingly, many of the most effective and well-known myths or claims about the Affordable Care Act (ACA) center on whether the law limits those choices. Attacks on the ACA charged that the law would reduce consumer choice in selection of health insurance plans, limit choice in physicians, and lead to one-size-fits-all health insurance benefits packages. One conservative think tank published a "top 10" list of the ways the ACA would curb consumer choice, writing that "Obamacare limits patient choice through expansive federal regulation of the insurance market, government interference in the decisions patients make with their doctors, and increased dependence on government health programs" (Nix, 2012). Some of these claims have been proven true, such as the Obama Administration's initial promise that individuals who were satisfied with their health insurance plans could keep those plans, while others have not been borne out. In general, the ACA does not appear to be limiting choices—especially for those who were previously uninsured.

A second, but related, line of attack on the law centered on rationing. Perhaps the most famous myth propagated on the rationing dimension (that has been repeatedly debunked since its inception) was the purported inclusion of "death panels" in the ACA. While this particular myth is an extreme example of how far the rationing claim can be used as a scare tactic, there are a number of other less blatant examples that Republicans used during the health reform debate—and continue to use—to raise concerns about the law. For instance, the role of comparative effectiveness research (CER), which aims to identify the relative effectiveness of different medical treatments to improve health outcomes and reduce spending on less beneficial treatments, has come under fire from conservatives and industry players who charge it will lead to rationing of health care services. This chapter examines the data and evidence underlying the claims surrounding the ACA's impact on consumer choice.

Q13. WERE PEOPLE SATISFIED WITH THEIR INSURANCE POLICIES ABLE TO KEEP THOSE POLICIES UNDER THE AFFORDABLE CARE ACT?

Answer: Not in all cases, despite repeated reassurances to that effect by the Obama Administration. The regulatory reforms contained in the ACA rendered some pre-ACA insurance policies inoperable because they did not meet new coverage parameters. Some insurance policies were subsequently canceled because they simply did not meet the law's requirements. People carrying these policies thus had to obtain new coverage.

The Facts: One of the most well-known claims about the ACA was that individuals satisfied with their coverage would be able to retain it. This was an oft-repeated promise made prior to and after the passage of the law—especially by the Obama Administration. The Administration stated (or implied) on 37 separate occasions from June 2009 to October 2013 that individuals who had health insurance would not have to change their coverage (Jacobson, 2013). The claim that individuals who liked their health insurance plans would be able to keep them drew criticism from many corners. Republicans, in particular, seized on these assurances as evidence that the ACA was being advanced under false pretenses. For instance, Rep. Tom Price (R-GA) stated in a weekly GOP address that "if you read the bill, that just isn't so. For starters, within five years, every health care plan will have to meet a new federal definition for coverage—one that your current plan might not match, even if you like it" (Price, 2009).

In 2013, insurers began to send notices to individuals whose policies were slated to be canceled because they did not meet the ACA's new minimum coverage requirements. Some estimates suggested that 2–2.6 million policies were slated to be canceled (CBS News, 2013; Clemans-Cope and Anderson, 2014). The plan cancellation notices were sent at the same time that HealthCare.gov was experiencing severe technical difficulties—calling into question whether individuals with canceled plans would be able to enroll in exchange coverage at all. As controversy over the plan cancellations mounted, the Administration issued a regulation allowing states to permit insurers to continue to sell these policies through October 1, 2016. The solution was largely a political one as it became clear that the Administration's promise that anyone who was satisfied with his or her existing plans would be able to keep them was impossible to uphold.

A primary goal of the ACA was to reform the individual insurance market—where people who were not covered by employer-sponsored insurance and who were ineligible for Medicare, Medicaid, or other sources of public coverage could choose a plan. In the individual market, insurers had the option of rejecting coverage for individuals with preexisting conditions, or not renewing coverage. In addition, there were no uniform rules for the types of benefits or services that had to be offered in an individual insurance market policy. For instance, around the time that the ACA was passed, 62 percent of individual market enrollees did not have coverage for maternity care, 34 percent did not have coverage for substance abuse services, 18 percent did not have coverage for mental health services, and 9 percent had no prescription drug coverage (Department of Health and Human Services, 2011).

The ACA included insurance market reforms to provide all people in the individual insurance market a basic package of benefits—termed essential health benefits (EHBs). Also, insurers had to adhere to new rules of conduct, such as no longer denying coverage for a preexisting condition or eliminating annual and lifetime benefit limits.

Some market reforms contained in the Affordable Care Act, such as allowing individuals up to age 26 to remain on their parents' coverage, went into effect in 2010; however, the ACA was written so that many of the most significant ones, such as the prohibition against denying coverage for preexisting conditions, did not go into effect until January 1, 2014, when the individual mandate went into effect and the health insurance exchanges launched. The new plans that were sold in the individual and small group markets (on and off the exchanges) had to adhere to the new market reforms and the EHBs.

Issuers had three options for how to deal with existing, pre-ACA plans that were considered "noncompliant" with the new insurance market reforms and benefit package requirements. First, they could amend them so they became compliant and thus eligible to be sold on or off the exchanges. Second, some were deemed "grandfathered"—meaning that if they met certain benefit and cost parameters, they did not have to comply with the new reforms if individuals had the coverage prior to the passage of the ACA in March 2010. The third option is what caused the most controversy—in many cases insurers opted to cancel the policies that were noncompliant for business reasons, including low enrollment or high average cost for a plan (Clemans-Cope and Anderson, 2014).

While it is difficult to assess how many individuals received plan cancellation notices, one team of researchers estimated that 2.6 million were affected, about 19 percent of the all the individual market policies sold in the United States. Meanwhile, about 75 percent of individual market policyholders did not get a cancellation notice from their insurer (Clemans-Cope and Anderson, 2014).

Of those who received cancellation notices, approximately half were estimated to be eligible for tax credits or cost-sharing subsidies, which could have reduced their payment for insurance relative to the current market (Clemans-Cope and Anderson, 2014). A Families USA analysis estimated that only 0.6 percent of individuals below the age of 65 years would actually lose coverage because of the ACA reforms and also be ineligible for a tax credit (Families USA, 2013). However, the plan cancellations caught the attention of lawmakers—especially because they occurred during the HealthCare.gov website troubles. For instance, Sen. Lamar Alexander (R-TN) stated: "I looked up the White House website this morning—'if you like your plan you can keep it and you don't have to change a thing due to the health care law. . . .' In fact, the plan cancels millions of individual policies" (Boyer, 2013). So, even though a relatively small number of insured Americans was affected by plan cancellations, opponents of the law seized on the notices as another sign of the law's shortcomings. There are several reasons for the controversy that ensued. As open enrollment began on October 1, 2013, the website's serious difficulties could have left millions without coverage on January 1, 2014, if they were unable to obtain a tax credit and enroll in a plan. As a result, some people with coverage could have been left uninsured if their plans were canceled and HealthCare.gov was still malfunctioning. Politically, the cancellation notices contradicted the Administration's repeated promises that individuals could keep their coverage if they wanted. The President and senior advisors in his Administration stated this on multiple occasions. Starting in 2009, the President made statements such as "And if you like your insurance plan, you will keep it. No one will be able to take that away from you. It hasn't happened yet. It won't happen in the future" (White House, 2009).

To mitigate both the practical and political problems facing the administration, on November 14, 2013, the Center for Consumer Information and Insurance Oversight (CCIIO) gave state insurance commissioners the option to extend these canceled policies (CCIIO, 2013). In March 2014, CCIIO further extended the transitional policy option for two years, until October 1, 2016 (CCIIO, 2014). However, not all states implemented the option to transition the canceled policies beyond January 1, 2014.

One thing to keep in mind is that the ACA's health insurance exchanges build on the private insurance market—and insurers have always been free to modify or cancel their plans in response to market demands and dynamics. Even in the absence of the ACA, there is no mechanism to require that plans remain available to consumers. However, despite the Administration's regulatory actions extending the time frame in which people could maintain policies, the fact is that in some instances, people were not always able to keep their existing policies given the insurance market reforms and benefit requirements enacted as part of the ACA.

FURTHER READING

Boyer, D. 2013. "Was Rep. Joe Wilson Right? Proof Obama Made Health Care Promise 23 Times." *Washington Times*, November 5, 2013. http://www.washingtontimes.com/news/2013/nov/5/obama-repeatedly-promised-people-could-keep-their-/#ixzz3Raq3GIHf.

CBS News. 2013. "Obamacare: More Than 2 Million People Getting Booted from Existing Health Insurance Plans." Accessed December 29, 2014. http://www.cbsnews.com/news/obamacare-more-than-2-million-people-getting-booted-from-existing-health-insurance-plans/.

Center for Consumer Information and Insurance Oversight. 2013. "Letter to Insurance Commissioners on Market Transitional Policy." Accessed December 9, 2014. http://www.cms.gov/CCIIO/Resources/Letters/Downloads/commissioner-letter-11-14-2013.PDF.

Center for Consumer Information and Insurance Oversight. 2014. "Insurance Standards Bulletin Series—Extension of Transitional Policy through October 1, 2016." Accessed December 9, 2014. http://www.cms.gov/CCIIO/Resources/Regulations-and-Guidance/Downloads/transition-to-compliant-policies-03-06-2015.pdf.

Clemans-Cope, L., and Anderson, N. 2014. "How Many Nongroup Policies Were Canceled? Estimates from December 2013?" *HealthAffairs Blog*, March 3, 2014. Accessed December 5, 2014. http://healthaffairs.org/blog/2014/03/03/how-many-nongroup-policies-were-canceled-estimates-from-december-2013/.

Department of Health and Human Services, Assistant Secretary for Planning and Evaluation. 2011. "Essential Health Benefits: Individual Market Coverage." Accessed December 29, 2014. http://kaiserfamily foundation.files.wordpress.com/2013/01/ib.pdf.

Families USA. 2013. "How Does the Affordable Care Act Affect People Who Buy Health Insurance in the Individual Market?" Accessed December 9, 2014. http://familiesusa.org/product/how-does-affordable-care-act-affect-people-who-buy-health-insurance-individual-market.

Jacobson, L. 2013. "Barack Obama Says That What He'd Said Was You Could Keep Your Plan 'If It Hasn't Changed since the Law Passed.'" Accessed November 6, 2014. http://www.politifact.com/truth-o-meter/statements/2013/nov/06/barack-obama/barack-obama-says-what-hed-said-was-you-could-keep/.

Nix, K. 2012. "Ten Ways Obamacare Limits Patient Choice." Heritage Foundation. Accessed December 30, 2014. http://www.heritage.org/research/reports/2012/07/10-ways-obamacare-limits-patient-choice.

Price, T. 2009. "Weekly GOP Address." Accessed November 6, 2014. https://www.youtube.com/watch?v=hBr3VcJ7v4M.

The White House. 2009. "Remarks by the President at the Annual Conference of the American Medical Association." Accessed February 12, 2015. http://www.whitehouse.gov/the-press-office/remarks-president-annual-conference-american-medical-association.

Q14. DID THE AFFORDABLE CARE ACT CONTAIN PROVISIONS FOR "DEATH PANELS"?

Answer: No. This specious assertion was roundly denounced as a particularly noxious example of political fearmongering, but it still colored the debate over the ACA. According to the death panel myth, the ACA included provisions creating death panels that would force Medicare beneficiaries to attend a counseling session on how to end their life, or suggested that government bureaucrats would be empowered with the authority to decide who would be eligible to receive care and who would be blocked from receiving life-saving medical care. The myth emerged in the summer of 2009, when health reform negotiations were in full force in the House and Senate, and quickly gained steam. When Congress adjourned for the summer August recess, lawmakers on both sides of the aisle were confronted at town hall meetings across the country with protesters angry about the so-called death panels in the health reform law. Scholars believe that the origin of the myth was a provision in the House health reform legislation—America's Affordable Health Choices Act of

2009—that would reimburse providers for voluntary advanced care planning consultations every five years (Fleming, 2009). This free end-of-life planning benefit was removed from the House bill when the death panel charge became a distraction, and it was not included in the final ACA.

The Facts: The "death panel" myth originated with House Tri-Committee legislation, called the Affordable Health Choices Act of 2009 or HR 3200, that included a provision that would pay physicians, nurse practitioners, or physician assistants to engage in voluntary advanced care planning consultations with Medicare beneficiaries (Fleming, 2009). The consultations could take place every five years and would cover questions and considerations for Medicare beneficiaries as they faced health challenges, would suggest people to speak with as part of advanced care planning, and would provide an explanation of advance directives, living wills, durable powers of attorney, and how they are used (Fleming, 2009). It is worth noting that the idea of coverage for advanced care planning consultations was not new—or partisan. A 2007 bill—"The Medicare End of Life Planning Act of 2007"—had three Republican cosponsors and would have provided payment to providers to perform the same services for Medicare beneficiaries (S.466, 2007).

The most prominent voices to initiate charges that these services might actually have sinister overtones were conservative writer (and former New York lieutenant governor) Elizabeth McCaughey and Sarah Palin. McCaughey made the death panel allegation for the first time on former Senator Fred Thompson's radio show on July 9, 2009, stating,

> And one of the most shocking things I found in this bill . . . where the Congress would make it mandatory—absolutely require—that every five years, people in Medicare have a required counseling session that will tell them how to end their life sooner, how to decline nutrition, how to decline being hydrated, how to go in to hospice care. And by the way, the bill expressly says that if you get sick somewhere in that five-year period—if you get a cancer diagnosis, for example—you have to go through that session again. (Dreier and Parker, 2009; NPR, 2009)

These statements set off a firestorm in the coming weeks, especially after former Alaska Governor and 2008 Republican Vice-Presidential candidate Sarah Palin issued a Facebook post alleging that the health reform legislation in Congress included death panels (Palin, 2009):

> The Democrats promise that a government health care system will reduce the cost of health care, but as the economist Thomas Sowell

has pointed out, government health care will not reduce the cost; it will simply refuse to pay the cost. And who will suffer the most when they ration care? The sick, the elderly, and the disabled, of course. The America I know and love is not one in which my parents or my baby with Down Syndrome will have to stand in front of Obama's "death panel" so his bureaucrats can decide, based on a subjective judgment of their "level of productivity in society," whether they are worthy of health care. Such a system is downright evil. (Palin, 2009)

McCaughey then followed up with op-eds in the *New York Post*, falsely alleging that physicians in the Obama Administration and working on health reform sought to give government the power to make health care decisions for individuals (McCaughey, 2009). An analysis tracing the spread of the death panel myth shows that it was quickly discussed on prominent conservative talk shows, including *The Sean Hannity Show*, *The Laura Ingraham Show*, and *The Rush Limbaugh Show* (Nyhan, 2010). From there, it spread to members of Congress, with House Minority Leader John Boehner issuing a press release on July 23, 2009, in which he warned that the voluntary advanced planning provision could result in "government-encouraged euthanasia" (Holan, 2009).

After this point, the death panel myth gained even more ground. As Congress adjourned in August 2009 and members of Congress returned home, town halls across the country filled with constituents convinced that the health reform legislation being considered in Congress contained such a provision. For instance, *The Economist* stated in August 2009 that members of Congress were being confronted at town hall meetings with the "outrageous allegation" (*The Economist*, 2009).

Although numerous media outlets and expert opinions debunked the myth, it remained a problem for the Obama Administration and other health reform advocates, in part because some conservative media outlets continued to devote time and space to the spurious charge. Even well-respected Republican health care experts such as Gail Wilensky lamented that the debate was focused on "red herrings" such as death panels (Rutenberg and Harris, 2009). In the end, the ACA did not include a provision providing payment for voluntary advanced care planning for Medicare beneficiaries because it seemed the only way to put the death panel myth to rest.

FURTHER READING

Dreier, H., and Parker, D. 2009. "Media echo Serial Misinformer McCaughey's False End-of-Life Counseling Claim." Accessed December 9, 2014.

http://mediamatters.org/research/2009/07/31/media-echo-serial-mis informer-mccaugheys-false/152759.

The Economist. 2009. "The Politics of Health Reform: Friend or Foe?" Accessed December 12, 2014. http://www.economist.com/node/14222 289?story_id=14222289.

Fleming, C. 2009. "Fact or Fiction: Advance Care Planning in Health Reform." *HealthAffairs Blog*, September 7, 2009. Accessed December 9, 2014. http://healthaffairs.org/blog/2009/09/07/fact-or-fiction-advance-care-planning-in-health-reform/.

Holan, A. 2009. "PolitiFact's Lie of the Year: 'Death Panels.'". Accessed December 12, 2014. http://www.politifact.com/truth-o-meter/article/2009/dec/18/politifact-lie-year-death-panels/.

McCaughey, Betsy. 2009. "Deadly Doctors." *New York Post*, July 24, 2009. Accessed December 12, 2014. http://nypost.com/2009/07/24/deadly-doctors/.

NPR. 2009. "Kill Grandma? Debunking a Health Bill Scare Tactic." Accessed December 9, 2014. http://www.npr.org/templates/story/story.php?storyId=111729363.

Nyhan, B. 2010. "Why the 'Death Panel' Myth Wouldn't Die: Misinformation in the Health Care Reform Debate." The Forum: The Politics of Health Care Reform, 8, 1, Article 5. Accessed December 12, 2014. http://www.dartmouth.edu/~nyhan/health-care-misinformation.pdf.

Palin, S. 2009. "Statement on the Current Health Care Debate." Accessed December 9, 2014. https://www.facebook.com/notes/sarah-palin/state menton-the-current-health-care-debate/113851103434.

Rutenberg, J., and Harris, G. 2009. "Conservatives See Need for Serious Health Debate." *New York Times*, September 2, 2009. Accessed December 12, 2014. http://www.nytimes.com/2009/09/03/health/policy/03 conservatives.html.

S.466. 2007. "The Medicare End of Life Choices Act of 2007." 110th Congress.

Q15. WILL THE AFFORDABLE CARE ACT'S NEW ENTITY ON COMPARATIVE EFFECTIVENESS RESEARCH LEAD TO RATIONING OF CARE?

Answer: No. Historically, Republicans as well as Democrats have regarded comparative effectiveness research (CER) as an important component of controlling costs and improving quality in health care in a way that does not harm individuals. Other industrialized nations have used CER to guide clinical decisions for years (Chalkidou and Anderson, 2009).

The Facts: The ACA established the Patient-Centered Outcomes Research Institute (PCORI) to conduct CER. CER builds evidence on the effectiveness, benefits, and potential risks of treatment options based on research that compares drugs, medical devices, tests, surgeries, or ways to deliver health care (AHRQ, 2014). PCORI is a nonprofit entity that receives funding from public and private sources to conduct CER; however, PCORI research on its own is not intended to be used to make coverage and payment decisions (Henry J. Kaiser Family Foundation, 2013).

PCORI's mission to conduct CER has garnered controversy since its legislative inception in 2007 and establishment in 2010. Opponents have expressed concerns that CER will be used to make coverage decisions that result in denying care to individuals—a phenomenon often referred to as "rationing." Rationing concerns were a key part of debate on health reform with GOP amendments filed to the Senate Health, Education, Labor and Pensions Committee (HELP) and Senate Finance Committee health reform bills prohibiting CER to be used to make coverage decisions—or stripping funding for the entity altogether (Patel, 2010). After the law was enacted, conservative analyses continue to suggest that PCORI could lead to rationing of care (Nix, 2012). However, there has been no indication that any of PCORI's research has resulted in a change in coverage decisions for payers, but the charges levied against it are more politically motivated attempts to maintain opposition to the law—and in some cases due to industry wariness of CER itself.

Even in the United States the concept of CER (and the controversy associated with it) is not new. As early as the 1990s, the Office of Technology Assessment, a former Congressional research support agency, discussed the objectives and hurdles associated with CER (Chalkidou and Anderson, 2009). CER has also not historically been a partisan issue. For instance, during the 2008 Presidential campaign, the Republican nominee—Sen. John McCain (R-AZ)—expressed support for CER (Commonwealth Fund, 2008). He advocated for a private-sector approach in which research findings would not necessarily be applied to Medicare benefit design (Commonwealth Fund, 2008). International CER activity, long-standing interest by policymakers in the United States, and bipartisan support for at least the concept would not have suggested that PCORI would be as controversial as it was during (and after) the health reform debate.

The discussions that eventually led to PCORI began in 2007 as Democrats took control of Congress and began working on reauthorization of the Children's Health Insurance Program (CHIP) and preparing for the potential of health reform. In response to a request by Senators Baucus (D-MT) and Conrad (D-ND), Congressional Budget Office (CBO) produced a report on CER, options for expanding the federal government's role in CER, and the potential impacts on federal health spending from expanded CER in the near- and long term (Congressional Budget Office, 2007). In general, experts agreed that CER could be a tool to address problems with quality and efficiency in health care by integrating evidence on the effectiveness of treatments and services into the care people received (Patel, 2010).

However, there was disagreement on what the federal role in CER should be as health reform began to take shape—especially between the House and the Senate. During CHIP reauthorization, House Democrats introduced creating a new CER center at the Agency for Healthcare Research and Quality. While the House CHIP reauthorization did not become law, it became the template for how CER would be included in the House health reform legislation in 2009. In the Senate, Democrats—led by Senators Baucus (D-MT) and Conrad (D-ND)—took a different approach. Their legislation, the Comparative Effectiveness Research Act of 2008 (S.3408), would establish a new public-private institute to conduct CER. In the end, the Baucus–Conrad approach was the one adopted in the ACA and eventually became PCORI.

Opponents of health reform promptly claimed that government-funded CER would lead to rationing care as information about the relative effectiveness of treatments, drugs, devices, and delivery approaches was produced. A number of prominent Republican leaders, including then House Minority Leader Boehner (R-OH), Representative Price (R-GA), who is also a physician, and Senators Kyl (R-AZ) and Roberts (R-KS), were strong critics of CER (Iglehart, 2010). Allegations that CER would lead to greater government control and rationing were also made during the summer of 2009 town halls and by prominent conservatives, such as George Will (Iglehart, 2010). Concerns have persisted that CER in the United States will lead to rationing the care that patients receive despite a lack of evidence that this has been the case. One conservative analyst wrote:

Regrettably, the PPACA puts CER use on the wrong path. Allowing unelected officials to determine how and to whom resources are allocated rather than empowering doctors and patients to make decisions is the wrong approach. Though the PPACA may not immediately result in overt rationing of care, its changes in Medicare open the door to top-down use of CER and interference with the care seniors receive.

As Medicare spending rises, PCORI and the research it produces will increasingly be considered a viable resource to micromanage the practice of medicine, and the PPACA creates the machinery to make this happen. For these reasons, the step forward should be to repeal the law and start over. (Nix, 2012)

PCORI became another provision to link health reform to future rationing of health care services—especially for seniors.

During the health reform debate, Republicans tried to amend the law to severely limit CER and its uses. On the first day of the HELP Committee markup, twenty amendments to change or eliminate the new CER entity proposed were made (Patel, 2010). For instance, Senator Enzi (R-WY) stated that the CER entity in AHRQ created in the Democratic Senate HELP Committee legislation would dictate what treatments to pay for (Patel, 2010). However, the HELP Committee legislation stated that any CER results were not coverage or cost mandates. Meanwhile, the Baucus–Conrad approach continued to be negotiated and was included in the Senate Finance Committee legislation. Here too, the concept was inundated with amendments to limit its scope or eliminate PCORI altogether.

In the end, PCORI was established as part of the ACA. PCORI's stated goal is to "close the gaps in evidence needed to improve key health outcomes . . . we identify critical research questions, fund patient-centered comparative clinical effectiveness research, or CER, and disseminate the results in ways that the end-users of our work will fund useful and valuable" (Patient Centered Outcomes Research Institute, 2014). Senator Baucus (D-MT) described PCORI's goals, the restrictions it operated under, and how it was unique in its construction:

> The goals of comparative effectiveness research and the new health reform law are the same: Both are about making the health system more effective and efficient for patients. . . .
>
> America produces the most technologically-advanced medical care in the world. Doctors and patients have more tests and treatment options to choose from than ever before. But in many cases, doctors and patients simply don't have enough reliable evidence to help us choose among the options. . . . The new health reform law fosters research that will help doctors and patients make the best

treatment decisions at the point of care. The law creates an independent institute—the "Patient Centered Outcomes Research Institute"—that will commission relevant, credible, unbiased research.

The new health reform law fosters research that will help doctors and patients make the best treatment decisions at the point of care. The law creates an independent institute—the "Patient Centered Outcomes Research Institute"—that will commission relevant, credible, unbiased research. . . . Institute will not develop medical guidelines, treatment protocols or coverage recommendations of any sort. The doctor-patient relationship is [sacred]. This research will not change that relationship in any way. Rather, it will serve to strengthen it. The law is clear: The purpose of the Institute is solely to generate useful information. By evaluating and comparing what works best, patients and providers can make better-informed decisions about care. . . .

Thus the Institute will be characterized by strong patient representation, a focus on patient outcomes, transparency, and a focused scope. All these features put the needs of patients first. We set out to develop a uniquely American approach. This is not Canada. This is not Britain. This is America. And we came up with a uniquely American solution. We put patients at the center of health care. (Baucus, 2010)

Despite a history of bipartisan support, and agreement among experts that CER had the potential to improve quality and could reduce costs over the long term, PCORI and its mission became controversial in the context of health reform. The charges of rationing that continued to be made against PCORI are largely politically motivated (and economically motivated in some cases where CER could impact industry) and aim to maintain opposition to the law by raising concerns about individual choice in health care.

FURTHER READING

Agency for Health Care Research and Quality (AHRQ). 2014. "What Is Comparative Effectiveness Research?" Accessed December 15, 2014. http://effectivehealthcare.ahrq.gov/index.cfm/what-is-comparative-effectiveness-research1/.

Baucus, M. 2010. "Baucus Remarks before the Partnership to Improve Patient Care Forum." Senate Finance Committee. Accessed February 22, 2015. http://www.finance.senate.gov/newsroom/chairman/rele ase/?id=67efbe3e-7686-4349-817b-5b0936606284.

Chalkidou, K., and Anderson, G. 2009. "Comparative Effectiveness Research: International Experiences and Implications for the United States." AcademyHealth, July 2009. Accessed December 17, 2014. http://www.academyhealth.org/files/publications/CER_International_Experience_09%20%283%29.pdf.

Commonwealth Fund. 2008. "Presidential Candidates' Health Reform Plans: Prospects for Promoting a High Performance Health System." Accessed December 23, 2014. http://www.commonwealthfund.org/publications/newsletters/states-in-action/2008/apr/april-may-2008/federal-activity/presidential-candidates-health-reform-plans--prospects-for-promoting-a-high-performance-health-syste.

Congressional Budget Office. 2007. "Research on the Comparative Effectiveness of Medical Treatments: Issues and Options for an Expanded Federal Role." Accessed December 23, 2014. http://www.cbo.gov/sites/default/files/12-18-comparativeeffectiveness.pdf.

Dentzer, S. 2010. "Comparative Effectiveness: Coherent Health Care at Last?" *Health Affairs*, 33, 12: 1756.

Henry J. Kaiser Family Foundation. 2013. "Summary of the Affordable Care Act." Accessed December 15, 2014. http://kff.org/health-reform/fact-sheet/summary-of-the-affordable-care-act/.

Iglehart, J. 2010. "The Political Fight over Comparative Effectiveness Research." *Health Affairs*, 29, 10: 1757–1760.

Nix, K. 2012. "Comparative Effectiveness Research under Obamacare: A Slippery Slope to Health Care Rationing." Accessed December 12, 2014. http://www.heritage.org/research/reports/2012/04/comparative-effectiveness-research-under-obamacare-a-slippery-slope-to-health-care-rationing.

Patel, K. 2010. "Health Reform's Tortuous Route to the Patient-Centered Outcomes Research Institute." *Health Affairs*, 29, 10, 1777–1782.

Patient Centered Outcomes Research Institute. 2014. "Why PCORI Was Created." Accessed December 23, 2014. http://www.pcori.org/content/why-pcori-was-created.

Q16. UNDER THE AFFORDABLE CARE ACT, DO INDIVIDUALS HAVE MORE LIMITED CHOICES IN THE PHYSICIANS THEY SEE FOR MEDICAL CARE?

Answer: This concern has proven true in some cases. An unintended consequence of the ACA is that individuals who have enrolled in health insurance exchange plans and in Medicaid may not truly have their choice of provider, albeit for different reasons.

The Facts: Consumer choice—in insurers, treatments, and physicians—is a main point of contention with the ACA. From the beginning of the health reform debate, opponents claimed that the national health reform proposals being advanced by Democrats would limit physician choice by restricting access, decreasing provider payments, or simply increasing wait times by providing more people with access to insurance (Tanner, 2014). On the other hand, the Obama Administration stated repeatedly that individuals who like their doctors would be able to keep them before and after the ACA was passed (Sebelius, 2010; The White House, 2009a, 2009b).

In 2014, when the Medicaid expansion and the health insurance exchanges launched, whether or not individuals truly had access to the physicians of their choice (or if they were losing choice in providers) could be assessed. For those enrolling in Medicaid and the exchanges, limited choice of providers—physicians, hospitals, and others—has been one of the main stories emerging from the types of coverage the newly insured are gaining. Early data indicate that insurers have created narrower networks, thereby limiting provider choice (Corlette, Lucia, and Ahn, 2014). On the other hand, there is no evidence that the majority of Americans with insurance—87 percent of the population—have had their choices limited as a result of the ACA (Smith and Medalia, 2014).

First, the market dynamics in the exchanges have placed pressures on insurers to price premiums competitively. One lever for competitive premium pricing is to create narrow provider networks. Narrow network products are effectively a tradeoff for consumers between premium price and choice of providers, including hospitals and physicians. In fact, narrow networks have a long history as a cost-containment mechanism dating back to the 1990s (Blumenthal, 2014). A recent six-state analysis found that in most cases, price was the determining factor for whether a provider was included in a network—not necessarily quality or patient outcomes (Corlette, Lucia, and Ahn, 2014). The analysis also found that insurers changed the provider networks for many of their plans after the ACA passed—so individuals may have found that their new plans did not allow them to remain with their previous providers (Corlette, Lucia, and Ahn, 2014). However, it does not appear that the ACA has directly led to more limited provider choice outside of the exchanges and Medicaid.

For different reasons, provider choice (especially physicians) is also limited for Medicaid beneficiaries—including those who became newly eligible as a result of the expansion. Physician surveys have consistently demonstrated that low Medicaid payment rates discourage them from seeing Medicaid patients (Henry J. Kaiser Family Foundation, 2014). The Government Accountability Office (GAO) also found that provider participation in Medicaid was problematic, with over two-thirds of states reporting difficulty ensuring sufficient numbers of Medicaid providers to serve beneficiaries (GAO, 2012). The reasons cited were Medicaid payment rates and general provider shortages as well (GAO, 2012). As a result, many Medicaid beneficiaries are unable to see any physician they want because physician participation in the program is often variable or limited.

Conservative think tanks have written extensively about the ACA resulting in restricted access to physicians, and GOP members of Congress have also highlighted that the ACA will lead to narrow networks (Senate Republican Policy Committee, 2013; Tanner, 2014). A Cato Institute commentary estimated that a majority of insurance plans post-ACA have fewer physicians and hospitals in their networks than prior to the ACA (Tanner, 2014). The commentary also referenced that Medicaid payment rates are often below provider costs—again, discouraging participation in the program and limiting provider choice (Tanner, 2014). Further politicizing the issue, the Senate Republican Policy Committee released policy briefs underscoring the concern that policies sold in the exchanges would have to restrict provider networks in order to remain price competitive, stating in one: "The truth is that President's health care law restricts people's ability to choose the provider or hospital that meets their needs" (Senate Republican Policy Committee, 2013). Some of these commentaries have been borne out—that exchange plans tend to have narrower provider networks and that low provider payment rates discourage participation in Medicaid; however, this does not necessarily translate to people's health care needs not being met.

Prior to health reform and since its passage, the Obama Administration strongly asserted that individuals will continue to have their choice of doctors. In 2009, during the debate over health reform President Obama stated to the American Medical Association: "If you like your doctor, you will be able to keep your doctor, period" (The White House, 2009a). Since, similar statements have been made, including by former Secretary of Health and Human Services Kathleen Sebelius. In a 2010 White House blog post, she made a similar assertion on provider choice (Sebelius, 2010). Individuals in exchange plans and Medicaid beneficiaries do not have unrestricted access to providers. For many with commercial insurance before the ACA, their new plans may include different providers in the network, forcing them to choose new physicians or hospitals.

At the same time, there are other important tradeoffs to consider, including what consumers in the new marketplaces value. To start, an estimated 8 million individuals gained insurance through the 2014 open enrollment alone (Long et al., 2014). For those who became newly insured, they may have had little to no access to providers and routine health care previously. A national poll in 2014 found that among those who were uninsured or purchasing coverage on the individual market before 2014, 54 versus 35 percent preferred less costly narrow network plans rather than plans with broader networks and higher premiums (Hamel, Firth, and Brodie, 2014). Narrow network products were 13 to 17 percent less expensive on average than broader network products and the majority of exchange enrollees purchased these products (Day, 2014; McKinsey Center for U.S. Health Reform, 2014). Another contributing factor to narrow networks may be provider consolidation—as health systems align with and purchase physician group practices or merge systems, there could be less provider choice. In the case of the narrow network products in the exchanges, issuers may be responding to consumer preferences and priorities—namely lower-priced plans that sacrifice broad networks.

On the other hand, 55 percent of those surveyed with employer coverage—who are most likely to not bear the full cost of their insurance—reported preferring costlier, broader network policies (Hamel, Firth, and Brodie, 2014). However, there is no indication that the ACA is leading to narrower networks for employer plans—as many employers were already turning to narrower networks to control costs separately from the ACA. While the ACA does not limit provider choice intentionally, the practical and competitive impacts of the exchanges and Medicaid expansion are to create narrower networks and more limited provider choice.

FURTHER READING

Blumenthal, D. 2014. "Reflecting on Health Reform—Narrow Networks: Boon or Bane?" Commonwealth Fund. Accessed May 13, 2015. http://www.commonwealthfund.org/publications/blog/2014/feb/narrows-networks-boon-or-bane.

Corlette, S., Lucia, K., and Ahn, S. 2014. "Implementation of the Affordable Care Act: Cross-Cutting Issues." Urban Institute. Accessed December 24, 2014. http://www.rwjf.org/content/dam/farm/reports/reports/2014/rwjf415649.

Day, R. 2014. "Exchanges and Narrow Networks—What Did Consumers Choose?" Accessed December 26, 2014. http://dayhealthstrategies.com/exchanges-and-narrow-networks-what-did-consumers-choose/.

Government Accountability Office (GAO). 2012. "Medicaid: States Made Multiple Program Changes, and Beneficiaries Generally Reported Access Comparable to Private Insurance." Accessed December 26, 2014. http://www.gao.gov/assets/650/649788.pdf.

Hamel, L., Firth, J., and Brodie, M. 2014. "Kaiser Health Tracking Poll: February 2014." Henry J. Kaiser Family Foundation. Accessed December 26, 2014. http://kff.org/health-reform/poll-finding/kaiser-health-tracking-poll-february-2014/.

Henry J. Kaiser Family Foundation. 2014. "Medicaid Moving Forward." Accessed December 26, 2014. http://kff.org/medicaid/fact-sheet/the-medicaid-program-at-a-glance-update/.

Long, S., Kenney, G., Zuckerman, S., Wissoker, D., Shartzer, A., Karpman, M., and Anderson, N. 2014. "QuickTake: Number of Uninsured Adults Continues to Fall under the ACA: Down by 8.0 Million in June 2014." Accessed December 26, 2014. http://hrms.urban.org/quicktakes/Number-of-Uninsured-Adults-Continues-to-Fall.html.

McKinsey Center for U.S. Health Reform. 2014. "Hospital Networks: Updated National View of Configurations on the Exchanges." Accessed December 26, 2014. http://healthcare.mckinsey.com/sites/default/files/McK%20Reform%20Center%20-%20Hospital%20networks%20national%20update%20%28June%202014%29_0.pdf.

Sebelius, K. 2010. "Keeping the Plan You Like." *The White House Blog.* Accessed December 24, 2014. http://www.whitehouse.gov/blog/2010/06/14/keeping-plan-you.

Senate Republican Policy Committee. 2013. "Obamacare Limits Patient Choice and Coverage." Accessed December 24, 2014. http://www.rpc.senate.gov/policy-papers/obamacare-limits-patient-choice-and-coverage.

Smith, J., and Medalia, C. 2014. "Health Insurance Coverage in the United States: 2013." Accessed U.S. Census Bureau. December 24, 2014. http://www.census.gov/content/dam/Census/library/publications/2014/demo/p60-250.pdf.

Tanner, 2014. "Obamacare: Fewer Doctors, More Demand." Cato Institute. Accessed December 24, 2014. http://www.cato.org/publications/commentary/obamacare-fewer-doctors-more-demand.

The White House. 2009a. "Remarks by the President at the Annual Conference of the American Medical Association." Accessed December 24, 2014. http://www.whitehouse.gov/the-press-office/remarks-president-annual-conference-american-medical-association.

The White House. 2009b. "Weekly Address: President Obama Says Health Care Reform Cannot Wait." Accessed December 24, 2014. http://www.whitehouse.gov/the_press_office/Weekly-Address-President-Obama-Says-Health-Care-Reform-Cannot-Wait/.

Q17. DO THE ESSENTIAL HEALTH BENEFITS REQUIREMENTS CONTAINED IN THE AFFORDABLE CARE ACT REQUIRE MORE COMPREHENSIVE COVERAGE TO BE MADE AVAILABLE TO CONSUMERS?

Answer: Yes, a key component of the insurance market reforms in the ACA is the Essential Health Benefits (EHB) requirements, which require all individual and small group market policies to provide a basic set of benefits starting in 2014. The EHBs include the following 10 categories of benefits:

- Ambulatory patient services (or outpatient services)
- Emergency services
- Hospitalization
- Prenatal, maternity, and newborn care
- Mental health and substance use disorder services
- Prescription drugs
- Rehabilitative and habilitative services and devices (services and devices to assist with injuries, disabilities, or chronic conditions to gain or recover skills)
- Laboratory services
- Preventive, wellness, and chronic disease management services
- Pediatric services (Health care.gov, 2014)

The Facts: The intent of the EHBs was to create a more standard floor for coverage across the nation so all individuals with insurance in the individual and small group markets had access to the same basic services, such as mental health and substance abuse services. For many—especially patient and consumer advocacy groups—this was a critical piece of health reform because many individuals and families—especially in the individual market—with health conditions could not get coverage that matched their health needs (Families USA, 2013b).

On the other hand, opponents of the ACA described the EHBs as a limitation on choice, and charged that they further concentrated decision making on health care in the hands of the federal government.

While not the most controversial part of the ACA, the EHBs have been linked to limiting individual and employer choice in benefit design (Hoff, 2011). There were also concerns that individuals satisfied with their current coverage would have to switch to plans that met the new coverage standards starting in 2014. Early evidence of the practical impact of the EHB requirements was observed in the fall of 2013, when cancellation notices were sent to an estimated 2–2.6 million Americans whose existing policies did not meet the new coverage requirements (CBS News, 2013; Clemans-Cope and Anderson, 2014).

Prior to the passage of the ACA, individual market plans varied widely from state to state in terms of the benefits they covered—with no national standard. Many plans did not offer the basic benefits listed earlier (Henry J. Kaiser Family Foundation, 2012). According to the Department of Health and Human Services (HHS), before the EHB package was required, 62 percent of individual market enrollees did not have coverage for maternity care, 34 percent did not have coverage for substance abuse services, 18 percent did not have coverage for mental health services, and 9 percent had no prescription drug coverage (Department of Health and Human Services, 2011). An industry study examined approximately 11,000 plans across the country and found that less than 2 percent met the EHB requirements—with maternity and pediatric care lacking most often, followed by substance use and mental health services (HealthPocket, 2013). The study also found that on average, plans covered 76 percent of the EHBs (HealthPocket, 2013). In terms of real impact, a 2009 survey found that 60 percent of respondents with health problems reported that it was difficult or impossible to find an insurance plan that covered their needs (Doty et al., 2009). The market incentives and dynamics in the individual insurance market in particular did not provide people with health problems with access to insurance plans that met their needs prior to 2014.

In response, the EHBs were included in health reform to provide a basic standard of coverage to those on the individual and small group markets, and to promote transparency by allowing consumers to compare coverage options more easily (Department of Health and Human Services, 2013). However, the attempt to create a national floor for individual and small group coverage for the first time was also viewed as a limitation on choice of plans and benefit designs, and as centralizing health care options and decision making at the federal level (Hoff, 2011). Hoff wrote:

> The Administration thus is given vast, but undefined, power to determine the care that must be covered by insurance plans. As a

practical matter, it will determine what kind of care is available to Americans who purchase insurance through the exchanges, how much the insurance will cost, and the extent of taxpayer subsidies. Whatever result it reaches will set a single standard—at least on paper—for everyone, despite the great variety of individual circumstances and desires. This is a fool's errand. A centralized authority cannot properly determine for every patient and every condition what must be provided, and when. But PPACA requires HHS to do just that. Its decisions will replace both individuals' choices and employers' judgments, and set the new contours of American health insurance. (Hoff, 2011)

While the ACA set the 10 general categories of benefits that had to be covered, HHS has left defining what the EHB package itself would include to states in the initial years of the insurance reform taking effect to avoid market disruption. There is likely to be more federal control and oversight over the EHBs over time, but at this time the federal government is not making coverage decisions over specific treatments, drugs, or medical devices.

An additional concern with the EHB approach was that requiring all individual market plans to comply with the benefit requirements would reduce consumer choice in terms of selecting a plan and benefit design that best met their needs. The alternative conservatives presented was to allow market competition and consumer choice to dictate benefit design and, thus, what plans would be sold (Haislmaier and Singer, 2013). However, the individual market previously was not responding to consumer. At this point, there is little evidence that the EHB coverage floor is limiting choice in benefit design for consumers; in fact, there seems to be more evidence that the EHB requirements are meeting consumer needs by providing coverage for basic services such as maternity care, pediatric care, and prescription drugs.

An additional criticism of the EHB requirements was that it would force individuals who were satisfied with their coverage to switch to new plans that were compliant with the coverage standards. This concern was partially borne out in the fall of 2013 when approximately 2–2.6 million individuals received cancellation notices for their policies, which were deemed noncompliant with the new ACA standards starting January 1, 2014 (CBS News, 2013; Clemans-Cope and Anderson, 2014). However, only 19 percent of individual market policyholders were estimated to receive a cancellation notice, and only 0.6 percent of individuals below 65 years of age were actually estimated to lose coverage because of the new requirements and also be ineligible for a tax credit (Clemans-Cope and Anderson, 2014; Families USA, 2013a). The practical impact of the EHB requirements on forcing consumers to switch plans they were satisfied with was not as significant as feared.

There were also concerns that the EHB requirements, which HHS will update periodically, would result in ever-rising coverage costs and complexity. First, opponents of this provision argued that special interests and lobbying to add more benefits or services to the EHB package during these periodic reviews would drive up costs over time, which has been borne out at the state level with pressures to include more services in state benefit mandates (Haislmaier, 2011; Nix, 2012). Second, the changing EHB packages would result in a "constantly" changing coverage mandates that insurers would have to comply with (Haislmaier, 2011). At least for 2014, there was evidence from an eight-state study that the burden on insurers was significant to come into compliance with the EHBs (Corlette, Monahan, and Lucia, 2013).

In the end, the EHB requirements create a new coverage floor for individuals who previously did not have access to basic benefits and care. While there are a number of intended and unintended consequences, it seems there is more evidence that the EHBs have expanded choice—in terms of the scope of coverage—available to those in the individual and small group markets, and at a minimum have not limited choice for most individuals. In addition, the federal government has ceded much of the decision making on the EHB package beyond the 10 categories of covered services to the states in the early years of the ACA, but has increased its oversight on the benefits consumers are purchasing in the individual market.

FURTHER READING

CBS News. 2013. "Obamacare: More Than 2 Million People Getting Booted from Existing Health Insurance Plans." Accessed December 29, 2014. http://www.cbsnews.com/news/obamacare-more-than-2-million-people-getting-booted-from-existing-health-insurance-plans/.

Clemans-Cope, L., and Anderson, N. 2014. "How Many Nongroup Policies Were Canceled? Estimates from December 2013?" *HealthAffairs Blog*, March 3, 2014. Accessed December 5, 2014. http://healthaffairs.org/blog/2014/03/03/how-many-nongroup-policies-were-canceled-estimates-from-december-2013/.

Corlette, S., Monahan, C., and Lucia, K. 2013. "Moving to High Quality, Adequate Coverage: State Implementation of New Essential Health Benefits Requirements." Robert Wood Johnson Foundation. Accessed

December 30, 2014. http://www.rwjf.org/content/dam/farm/reports/reports/2013/rwjf407484.

Department of Health and Human Services, Assistant Secretary for Planning and Evaluation. 2011. "Essential Health Benefits: Individual Market Coverage." Accessed December 29, 2014. http://kaiserfamily foundation.files.wordpress.com/2013/01/ib.pdf.

Department of Health and Human Services. 2013. "Health Care Law Allows Consumers to Easily Find and Compare Options Starting in 2014." Accessed December 29, 2014. http://www.hhs.gov/news/press/2013pres/02/20130220a.html.

Doty, M., Collins, S., Nicholson, J., and Rustgi, S. 2009. "Failure to Protect: Why the Individual Insurance Market Is Not a Viable Option for Most U.S. Families." Commonwealth Fund. Accessed December 29, 2014. http://www.commonwealthfund.org/~/media/Files/Publications/Issue%20Brief/2009/Jul/Failure%20to%20Protect/1300_Doty_failure_to_protect_individual_ins_market_ib_v2.pdf.

Families USA. 2013a. "How Does the Affordable Care Act Affect People Who Buy Health Insurance in the Individual Market?" Accessed December 9, 2014. http://familiesusa.org/product/how-does-affordable-care-act-affect-people-who-buy-health-insurance-individual-market.

Families USA. 2013b. 10 Essential Health Benefits Insurance Plans Must Cover Starting in 2014. Accessed December 29, 2014. http://familiesusa.org/blog/10-essential-health-benefits-insurance-plans-must-cover-starting-in-2014.

Haislmaier, E. 2011. "Obamacare and Insurance Benefit Mandates: Raising Premiums and Reducing Patient Choice." Heritage Foundation. Accessed December 30, 2014. http://www.heritage.org/research/reports/2011/01/obamacare-and-insurance-benefit-mandates-raising-premiums-and-reducing-patient-choice.

Haislmaier, E., and Singer, A. 2013. "Obamacare's Essential Benefits Regulation Creates Disparities among States." Accessed December 30, 2014. http://www.heritage.org/research/reports/2013/04/obamacare-s-essential-benefits-regulation-creates-disparities-among-states.

Health care.gov. 2014. "What Marketplace Health Plans Cover." Accessed December 29, 2014. https://www.health care.gov/coverage/what-marketplace-plans-cover/.

HealthPocket. 2013. "Almost No Existing Health Plans Meet New ACA Essential Health Benefit Standards." Accessed May 22, 2015. https://www.healthpocket.com/healthcare-research/infostat/few-existing-health-plans-meet-new-aca-essential-health-benefit-standards/#.VV9AU_lViko.

Henry J. Kaiser Family Foundation. 2012. "Essential Health Benefits: What Have States Decided for Their Benchmark?" Accessed December 29, 2014. http://kff.org/health-reform/fact-sheet/quick-take-essential-healt h-benefits-what-have-states-decided-for-their-benchmark/.

Hoff, J. 2011. "Implementing Obamacare: A New Exercise in Old-Fashioned Central Planning." Heritage Foundation. Accessed December 29, 2014. http://www.heritage.org/research/reports/2010/09/ implementing-obamacare-a-new-exercise-in-old-fashioned-central-planning?query=Implementing+Obamacare:+A+New+Exercise+ in+Old-Fashioned+Central+Planning.

Nix, K. 2012. "Ten Ways Obamacare Limits Patient Choice." Heritage Foundation. Accessed December 30, 2014. http://www.heritage.org/ research/reports/2012/07/10-ways-obamacare-limits-patient-choice.

Q18. WILL THE AFFORDABLE CARE ACT REDUCE THE NUMBER OF PRIVATE MEDICARE ADVANTAGE PLANS FOR SENIORS?

Answer: Unknown at this point in time. One of the mechanisms by which the ACA paid for itself was through reductions in payments to Medicare Advantage, which went into effect in 2011. Overall, plan participation in the program remained steady through 2014 and then decreased slightly in 2015 (Avalere Health, 2014). Most important, however, enrollment continued to grow in the program with a record 16 million beneficiaries in Medicare Advantage plans in 2015—6.3 million more than what CBO projected when the ACA passed in 2010 (Neuman and Jacobson, 2014). Early evidence does not suggest that the Medicare Advantage market is suffering on average across the country as a result of the ACA; however, many experts want to assess the longer-term impacts of the Medicare Advantage payment reductions before making any conclusive determinations.

The Facts: Medicare offers most beneficiaries the choice of enrolling in the traditional program, or in private Medicare Advantage plans. Private plans in Medicare are not new—they have been an option, albeit in different forms, for several decades (Henry J. Kaiser Family Foundation, 2014). In their earliest form in the 1970s, they were primarily Health Maintenance Organizations (HMOs), but by the 2000s they were more focused on expanding access to private plans and extra benefits (Henry J. Kaiser Family Foundation, 2014).

Today, Medicare's private managed care program is called Medicare Advantage. In 2014, the program served 16 million beneficiaries and paid

Medicare Advantage plans $156 billion (Congressional Budget Office, 2015). Leading up to health reform, there was growing concern about the costs of the Medicare Advantage program relative to traditional Medicare. In 2009, the Medicare Payment Advisory Commission (MedPAC) estimated that Medicare Advantage plans were overpaid 14 percent on average in comparison to traditional fee-for-service Medicare (Medicare Payment Advisory Commission, 2009). In response, architects of the ACA made significant changes to how Medicare Advantage plans were paid to bring spending in line with traditional Medicare. In total, the ACA reduced payments to Medicare Advantage plans by approximately $200 billion from 2010 through 2019 (Congressional Budget Office, 2010a).

The magnitude of cuts to private plans in Medicare was expectedly controversial. Critics charged that there would be fewer Medicare Advantage plans for seniors to choose from, that they would see a decline in benefits and higher premiums, and that more seniors would transition back into traditional Medicare, which has quality and efficiency issues of its own (Capretta, 2011). During the Senate floor debate on the ACA, prominent GOP Senators, including Minority Leader McConnell and Senate Finance Committee member Orrin Hatch, spoke at length about how the Medicare Advantage payment cuts would reduce benefits enrolled seniors receive, as well as limit plan choice (Congressional Record Senate, 2009). The debate on the impacts of the Medicare Advantage cuts continued, with the Republican Policy Committee reporting that seniors would face more limited plan choice, higher costs, and more limited provider choice (Republican Policy Committee, 2009).

The cost differential between traditional Medicare and Medicare Advantage was striking by the time the health reform debate was fully under way in 2009. The MedPAC is an independent Congressional agency with 17 bipartisan Commissioners overseeing its work. In March 2009, MedPAC reported that Medicare Advantage plan payments continued to be higher—114 percent on average—than what Medicare costs were for similar beneficiaries in the traditional program (Medicare Payment Advisory Commission, 2009). MedPAC concluded that the additional costs of Medicare Advantage, which were being completely financed by Medicare and beneficiaries, were contributing to the long-term insolvency of the program (Medicare Payment Advisory Commission, 2009). Another important observation was that quality varied across Medicare Advantage plans, with established HMO's tending to be high quality relative to new plans (Medicare Payment Advisory Commission, 2009). MedPAC's conclusions provided momentum to members in the House and Senate that sought to reform the program to both bring greater efficiency to Medicare Advantage and improve quality in the program as part of health reform.

Medicare Advantage plans are paid based on bids they submit to the Centers for Medicare and Medicaid Services. The plan bids are then compared to a "benchmark" based on a formula that varies by county. The benchmark sets the maximum allowable payment from Medicare. If a plan bid is higher than the benchmark, the Medicare beneficiaries must pay the difference through higher premiums. If a plan bid is lower than the benchmark, then the plan and Medicare split the difference and the plan must use its share of the difference to provide additional benefits to enrolled beneficiaries. The ACA essentially reduces these benchmarks so that they are closer to spending in the traditional Medicare program. In 2011, the benchmark was frozen at 2010 levels and further reductions are being phased in through 2016. The second critical change to Medicare Advantage in the ACA was a quality bonus program based on a five-star rating system for higher-quality plans through 2014. In total, CBO estimated approximately $200 billion in federal savings from 2010 to 2019 from the direct payment reductions to plans and other indirect impacts of the changes (Congressional Budget Office, 2010a).

The significant payment reductions and focus on improving quality for a program that served 10.5 million enrollees in 2009 quickly came under fire (Henry J. Kaiser Family Foundation, 2014). Critics contended that the payment reductions to Medicare Advantage plans would disrupt coverage for millions of seniors in the program by reducing coverage choices, eliminating benefits in Medicare Advantage, and increasing their costs (Capretta, 2011; Congressional Record, 2009; Republican Policy Committee, 2009). During the Senate floor debate, GOP leaders, including Minority Leader McConnell (R-KY), and Senators McCain (R-AZ), Alexander (R-TN), and Hutchison (R-TX) all cited that the payment reductions would result in reduced choice and benefits for beneficiaries. These concerns were rooted in the potential for political fallout from seniors if fewer Medicare Advantage plans were available (or benefits in those plans were reduced); however, the rhetoric was at least partially designed to mobilize seniors' opposition to the ACA itself. Minority Leader McConnell (R-KY) stated:

> Seniors do not want Senators fooling with Medicare. Let me say that again. Seniors do not want Senators fooling with Medicare. They want us to fix it, to strengthen it, to preserve it for future generations—not raid it like a giant piggy bank in order to create some entirely new government program . . . proponents of this

measure authorized $120 billion in cuts to Medicare Advantage and in the process they expressly voted to violate the President's pledge that seniors who like the plans they have can keep them. The President has said seniors who like the plans they have can keep them—because you can't cut $120 billion from a benefits program, obviously, without cutting benefits. (Congressional Record, 2009)

Bolstering this belief, CBO estimated that the payment reductions would lead to an estimated 5 million fewer beneficiaries in Medicare Advantage than previously projected (Congressional Budget Office, 2010b). Clearly, there was significant cause for concern that the Medicare Advantage program would be much more limited following the payment reductions. However, Medicare Advantage enrollment has outpaced original projections. In 2014, approximately 16 million individuals are expected to choose private plans—over 6 million more than what CBO projected after the ACA passed (Neuman and Jacobson, 2014). This trend is expected to continue despite the payment reductions.

Second, critics were concerned that Medicare Advantage plans would exit the market (Capretta, 2011). While the number of plans has remained fairly steady since the payment reductions went into effect

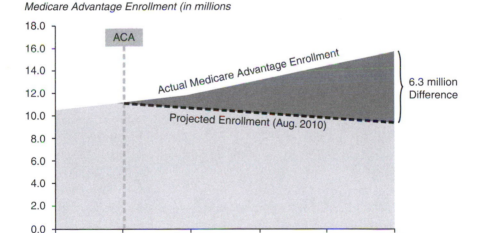

Medicare Advantage Enrollment (in millions

Figure 3.1 Actual versus Projected Medicare Advantage Enrollment, 2010–2014

Source: Neuman, T. and Jacobson, G. 2014. "Medicare Advantage: Take Another Look." Henry J. Kaiser Family Foundation. Accessed October 6, 2015. http://kff.org/medicare/perspective/medicare-advantage-take-another-look/

in 2011, only modest decreases were observed for the 2015 plan year (Avalere Health, 2014). An analysis by Avalere Health found that there was a 3 percent decrease in the numbers of plans participating in Medicare Advantage across the country in 2015 (Avalere Health, 2014). The consulting firm attributed the decrease in plan participation to reduced payment levels, low growth in benchmarks, and the end of the quality bonus program (Avalere Health, 2014). However, it still concluded that plan participation was largely stable across most of the United States with some geographic exceptions (Avalere Health, 2014). While the payment reductions to Medicare Advantage plans are still ongoing, there is little evidence to suggest that the program is failing—despite the political rhetoric about the damage the ACA would do to the benefits seniors received. In fact, growth is significantly outpacing projections, and plan participation is generally stable.

FURTHER READING

Avalere Health. 2014. "Avalere Analysis Reveals Significant Consolidation among PDPs."

Capretta, J. 2011. "Obamacare and Medicare Advantage Cuts: Undermining Seniors' Coverage Options." Heritage Foundation. Accessed December 30, 2014. http://www.heritage.org/research/reports/2011/01/obamacare-and-medicare-advantage-cuts-undermining-seniors-coverage-options.

Congressional Budget Office. 2010a. "Letter to the Honorable Nancy Pelosi on H.R. 4872, the Reconciliation Act of 2010. March 20, 2010." Accessed June 19, 2014. https://www.cbo.gov/sites/default/files/cbofiles/ftpdocs/113xx/doc11379/amendreconprop.pdf.

Congressional Budget Office. 2010b. "Selected CBO Publications Related to Health Care Legislation 2009–2010." Accessed December 30, 2014. http://www.cbo.gov/sites/default/files/12-23-selectedhealth carepublications.pdf.

Congressional Budget Office. 2015. "March 2015 Medicare Baseline." Accessed May 22, 2015. http://www.cbo.gov/sites/default/files/cbofiles/attachments/44205-2015-03-Medicare.pdf.

Congressional Record. 2009. "S12356. Congressional Record—Senate. December 4, 2009." Accessed December 30, 2014. http://www.gpo.gov/fdsys/pkg/CREC-2009-12-04/pdf/CREC-2009-12-04-pt1-PgS12356-4.pdf.

Henry J. Kaiser Family Foundation. 2014. "Medicare Advantage Fact Sheet." Accessed December 30, 2014. http://kaiserfamilyfoundation.files.wordpress.com/2014/05/2052-18-medicare-advantage.pdf.

Medicare Payment Advisory Commission. 2009. "Report to the Congress: Medicare Payment Policy." Accessed December 30, 2014. http://www .medpac.gov/documents/reports/mar09_ch03.pdf?sfvrsn=0.

Neuman, T. and Jacobson, G. 2014. "Medicare Advantage: Take Another Look." Henry J. Kaiser Family Foundation. Accessed October 6, 2015. http://kff.org/medicare/perspective/medicare-advantage-take-another-look/

Republican Policy Committee. 2009. "Obamacare Pounds Medicare Advantage." Accessed December 30, 2014. http://www.rpc.senate.gov/ policy-papers/obamacare-pounds-medicare-advantage.

Senate Finance Committee. 2009. "The Patient Protection and Affordable Care Act: Strengthening Medicare and Protecting Benefits for America's Seniors." Accessed December 30, 2014. http://www .finance.senate.gov/newsroom/chairman/release/?id=bd8bd091-d7de-48cb-a11b-300484dc11b9.

4

❖

Employer-Sponsored Insurance and the Affordable Care Act

Employer-sponsored insurance has been—and continues to be—the backbone of health insurance coverage in the United States. While the percentage of Americans receiving health insurance from their employers has been declining in recent years, the system still provides coverage to 149 million Americans—or approximately 50 percent of the population (Henry J. Kaiser Family Foundation and Health Research &Educational Trust, 2014). Given the breadth and general stability of this market, Democrats sought to craft a health reform law that would maintain, and even strengthen employer-sponsored insurance (especially for small businesses), as well as reduce job lock for those who remained in their jobs because insurance was inaccessible otherwise. There were both policy and political reasons for doing so. In terms of policy, the Affordable Care Act (ACA) sought to expand coverage to those who were uninsured—and not upend well-established coverage mechanisms. In terms of the politics, changes that would cause people to lose their employer-sponsored insurance would signal almost certain failure for a health reform effort—fears that people would lose their coverage would have led to widespread opposition.

Given how central employer-sponsored insurance is in the U.S. health care system, how the law impacts this coverage has been heavily debated. Republican members of Congress and conservative think tanks have charged that the ACA would result in millions of Americans losing employer-sponsored insurance. While there have been some changes in the employer-sponsored insurance market as a result of new coverage requirements and the launch of health insurance exchanges that are new mechanisms for obtaining insurance, the evidence to date suggests that employers are generally continuing to offer coverage to their employees. Another flashpoint on employer issues has been the employer coverage requirements—or "free-rider" provisions—that require employers of a certain size to provide affordable coverage or face penalties. Republicans have contended that these policies have had negative impacts on job growth and contributed to employer hesitation to hire new workers. For instance, Republican Governor Bobby Jindal (LA) stated, *"Why not delay all of the mandates in Obamacare [which] has become such a job killer in our economy"* (Kessler, 2014). This chapter examines the myths and claims surrounding the law's impacts on employer-sponsored insurance, such as whether or not it will lead (or has led) to widespread erosion of the market, if it actually promotes entrepreneurship by reducing job lock, as well as the costs and changes the law has placed on businesses.

Q19. WILL THE AFFORDABLE CARE ACT ACCELERATE THE EROSION OF EMPLOYER-SPONSORED INSURANCE IN AMERICA?

Answer: It is too early to tell. Because the primary goal of the ACA was to extend coverage to the uninsured, Congress focused on preserving employer-sponsored insurance in order to not disrupt coverage for the majority of working Americans. The ACA thus builds on and complements, rather than replaces, employer-sponsored insurance programs. And while employer-sponsored policies will remain the foundation of America's health insurance system for at least the near future, the ACA does provide health coverage options to would-be entrepreneurs who might otherwise be forced to remain with their employer for health insurance reasons.

The Facts: Employer-sponsored insurance is the foundation of our health insurance system. Approximately 50 percent of Americans—or an estimated 149 million individuals below the age of 65—receive health insurance coverage through an employer (Henry J. Kaiser Family Foundation and Health Research &Educational Trust, 2014). The goal of the ACA was to extend coverage to the uninsured and a basic level of coverage to those outside of the employer-sponsored insurance market. However, any changes to the availability and subsidization of coverage outside of the employer market could likely impact employer-sponsored benefits as well. Given the reach (and relative generosity) of employer-sponsored insurance, the architects of the ACA sought to build on the system of employer-sponsored insurance by including a number of policy provisions to—at a minimum—maintain this market.

How the ACA would affect employer-sponsored insurance over the short- and long term has been heavily debated—and will continue to be for some time. While some of the disagreement falls along party lines, there is also disagreement among researchers, consultants, and benefits experts about whether the ACA will result in significant erosion of employer-sponsored insurance. The highest estimates suggest that as many as 35 million Americans could move from employer-sponsored coverage as a result of the ACA (Holtz-Eakin and Smith, 2011). However, estimates from researchers who have constructed microsimulation models intended to project the impacts of changes in insurance on difference sources of coverage indicate relatively low to moderate levels of both increases and decreases in employer-sponsored insurance (Blumberg et al., 2012; Congressional Budget Office, 2014; Lewin Group, 2010; Eibner, Hussey, and Girosi, 2010). While the impacts of the ACA on employer-sponsored coverage will continue to unfold as implementation of the law continues, large-scale erosion in employer-sponsored insurance has not been observed—with some exceptions for certain populations of workers and firm types.

Employer-sponsored insurance became a primary mechanism for covering Americans due to a series of tax and other policy decisions dating back to the 1930s. The most critical policy decision occurred in the 1940s—to make employer-sponsored health insurance benefits tax exempt. This was one of the most significant factors in making employer-sponsored insurance becoming the foundation of health insurance coverage in the United States and planting the seed for much of today's system. Today, employer-sponsored insurance covers 149 million Americans below the age of 65—or approximately 50 percent of the U.S. population. (Henry J. Kaiser Family Foundation and Health Research &Educational Trust, 2014). Because the primary goal of the ACA was to extend coverage to the uninsured, Congress focused on preserving employer-sponsored insurance in order to not disrupt coverage for the majority of working Americans—and in essence building on the long-existing system.

Over the past several decades, employers have provided health insurance to employees for three primary reasons. Understanding how the

ACA could change the traditional reasons employers offer coverage is important to predicting what the future of the employer-based system is. First, health insurance for individuals and their families is a recruiting and retention tool to attract and maintain talent. Second, prior to the ACA, there was no guarantee of alternative coverage option that was affordable and that covered individuals regardless of preexisting conditions. Finally, having health insurance and access to medical care is thought to boot worker productivity. The ACA largely affects the second reason employers provide health insurance to workers by offering more-affordable coverage options and guaranteed access to coverage for a basic set of benefits due to the insurance market reforms in the law; however, the ACA does not affect the primary reasons employers offer health insurance—the need to recruit and retain talent (Avalere Health, 2011).

However, rising health care costs are also affecting employers and calling into question whether many can (or want to) continue to offer coverage. The new health insurance exchanges and subsidies for those with incomes below 400 percent of the Federal Poverty Level (FPL) provide new coverage options that would allow those with preexisting conditions to obtain insurance, a basic package of Essential Health Benefits (EHBs), and financial assistance for many—among other reforms. Some experts and private companies predicted that the ACA would lead to employers "dumping" or dropping coverage for their workers with the exchanges and the subsidies to purchase coverage. For instance, one analysis predicted that up to 35 million Americans could lose employer-sponsored insurance (Holtz-Eakin and Smith, 2011). The report reasoned that even with free-rider penalties in place to prevent large employers from dropping coverage, it would still be more cost-effective for many to stop offering health insurance coverage and pay the penalties (Holtz-Eakin and Smith, 2011). Upon closer inspection, many of the assumptions made in the paper were flawed and for many employers, dropping coverage may not be more cost-effective once penalties, taxes, and increasing wages to compensate for the loss in insurance are taken into account (Avalere Health, 2011; Blumberg et al., 2012). McKinsey & Company released one of the most controversial employer surveys released during this time, projecting that 30 percent of employers would definitely or probably stop offering coverage altogether; however, the survey methodology was criticized and the company clarified that its results were not meant to be predictive in nature (McKinsey & Company, 2011; Singhal, Steuland, and Ungerman, 2011). These studies and surveys predicting large-scale erosion of employer-sponsored insurance garnered significant media and political attention—and were regarded as a very negative unintended consequence of the law.

At the same time, a large body of research and employer surveys have regularly examined the potential impacts of the ACA on employer-sponsored insurance. Most have not predicted the level of erosion referenced earlier—although most indicate that some loss of employer-sponsored coverage will occur as the ACA is fully implemented. A handful of academic and think tank researchers, as well as the CBO, have created microsimulation models to predict the impact of policy changes and the ACA in particular on different forms of health insurance coverage using empirical data and evidence whenever possible. First, the CBO model most recently predicted that approximately 7 million people would lose employer-sponsored insurance (Congressional Budget Office, 2014). Other researchers, such as at the RAND Corporation, actually projected that employer-sponsored insurance would increase by 13 million (Eibner, Hussey, and Girosi, 2010). The Urban Institute's model also predicted a slight increase of 5 million individuals in employer coverage (Blumberg et al., 2012). The Lewin Group model predicted that 3 million fewer individuals would have employer-sponsored insurance following implementation of the ACA (Lewin Group, 2010). Finally, a survey-based study of labor unions and health policy experts also predicted general stability in employer-sponsored insurance over the near term—especially for middle- and higher-income workers who receive employer-sponsored insurance and that would not be eligible for subsidies (Reuther, 2011). In general, the microsimulation models tend to predict anywhere from low to moderate increases or decreases in employer-sponsored insurance and nowhere near the level of instability that the previously referenced studies and surveys reported.

In addition to the research models, employer surveys indicate a general stability in employer-sponsored insurance in the near- to mid-term. A 2014 Mercer employer survey found that 22 percent of respondents reported a likely increase in employer-sponsored insurance because of the requirement to offer coverage to those working 30 or more hours a week or face a penalty starting 2015 (Mercer, 2014). The 2014 Towers Watson survey reported that 87 percent of employers stated that health care benefits would be a "key part" of their employee benefits package in 2015 (Towers Watson, 2014). These annual surveys do not indicate major changes in the incentives to offer insurance for employers—even after the launch of the exchanges.

However, there is greater uncertainty about the provision of employer-sponsored insurance over the long run for a number of reasons. For instance, beginning in 2017, states have the option to allow employers with more than 100 workers to enter the exchanges, which could increase employers dropping coverage if the health insurance exchanges are successful and viable marketplaces. There are also particular firms for which it makes financial sense to drop coverage altogether. For instance, firms with lower-wage workers who will be eligible for subsidies or those with part-time or seasonal employment are going to be more likely to drop coverage (Avalere Health, 2011; Reuther, 2011). In addition, there is evidence that employers have begun to drop coverage for early retirees—instead giving many a fixed contribution to buy coverage through the exchanges (Fronstin and Adams, 2012; Reuther, 2011). While these subpopulations are experiencing changes in their coverage, large-scale erosion of employer-sponsored insurance is not being seen and is not anticipated in the near future.

FURTHER READING

Avalere Health. 2011. "The Affordable Care Act's Impact on Employer Sponsored Insurance: A Look at the Microsimulation Models and Other Analyses." Accessed January 8, 2015. http://www.avalerehealth .net/pdfs/2011-06-17_ESI_memo.pdf.

Blumberg, L., Buettgens, M., Feder, J., and Holahan, J. 2012. "Implications for the Affordable Care Act on American Business." Urban Institute. Accessed January 8, 2015. http://www.urban.org/Uploaded PDF/412675-Implications-of-the-Affordable-Care-Act-for-American-Business.pdf.

Congressional Budget Office. 2014. "Updated Estimates of the Effects of the Insurance Coverage Provisions of the Affordable Care Act, April 2014." Accessed January 8, 2015. http://www.cbo.gov/sites/default/files/45231-ACA_Estimates.pdf.

Eibner, C., Hussey, P., and Girosi, F. 2010. "The Effects of the Affordable Care Act on Workers' Health Insurance Coverage." *New England Journal of Medicine*, 363: 1393–1395.

Fronstin, P., and Adams, N. 2012. "Employment-Based Retiree Health Benefits: Trends in Access and Coverage 1997–2010." Employee Benefit Research Institute. Accessed January 8, 2015. http://www.ebri.org/pdf/briefspdf/ebri_ib_10-2012_no377_rethlth.pdf.

Henry J. Kaiser Family Foundation and Health Research Educational Trust. 2014. "Employer Health Benefits: 2014 Annual Survey." Accessed January 3, 2015. http://files.kff.org/attachment/2014-employer-heal th-benefits-survey-full-report.

Holtz-Eakin, D., and Smith, C. 2011. "Labor Markets and Health Care Reform: New Results." American Action Forum. Accessed January 7, 2015. http://americanactionforum.org/research/labor-markets-and-health-care-reform-new-results.

Kessler, G. 2014. "Is Obamacare a 'Job Killer'?" *Washington Post*, February 26, 2014. http://www.washingtonpost.com/blogs/fact-checker/wp/2014/02/26/is-obamacare-a-job-killer/.

Lewin Group. 2010. "Patient Protection and Affordable Care Act (PPACA): Long Term Costs for Governments, Employers, Families and Providers." Accessed January 8, 2015. http://www.lewin.com/~/media/lewin/site_sections/publications/lewingroupanalysis-patientprotectionandaffordablecareact2010.pdf.

McKinsey & Company. 2011. "Employer Survey on U.S. Health Care Reform: Details Regarding the Survey Methodology." Accessed January 8, 2015. http://www.mckinsey.com/features/us_employer_health care_survey.

Mercer. 2014. "Survey Predicts Health Benefit Cost Increases Will Edge Up in 2015." Accessed January 8, 2015. http://www.mercer.com/news room/survey-predicts-health-benefit-cost-increases-will-edge-up-in-2015-spurring-employers-to-take-action.html.

Reuther, A. 2011. "Workers and Their Health Care Plans: The Impact of New Health Insurance Exchanges and Medicaid Expansion on Employer-Sponsored Health Care Plans." Center for American Progress. Accessed January 8, 2015. http://cdn.americanprogress.org/wp-content/uploads/issues/2011/09/pdf/health_care_plans.pdf.

Singhal, S., Steuland, J., and Ungerman, D. 2011. "How U.S. Health Care Reform Will Affect Employee Benefits." McKinsey & Company. Accessed January 8, 2015. http://www.mckinsey.com/insights/health_systems_and_services/how_us_health_care_reform_will_affect_employee_benefits.

Towers Watson. 2014. "2014 Health Care Changes Ahead Survey Emerging Factors Influencing Employer-Sponsored Health Care Benefits." Accessed January 8, 2015. http://www.towerswatson.com/en-US/Insights/IC-Types/Survey-Research-Results/2014/09/2014-health-care-changes-ahead-survey-report.

Q20. IS THE AFFORDABLE CARE ACT A "JOB KILLER"?

Answer: Assertions that Obamacare would result in large-scale job losses have been proven mostly false in most areas of the economy, although data indicate that in a few low-wage industry sectors a modest negative impact has been felt.

The Facts: Health care spending accounts for approximately one-sixth of the U.S. Gross Domestic Product and is climbing (Centers for Medicare and Medicaid Services, 2014). As a result, any major piece of health care legislation inevitably affects the economy—and very often the labor market as well. This is because nearly half of Americans—149 million individuals below the age of 65—receive insurance through their employers (Henry J. Kaiser Family Foundation and Health Research &Educational Trust, 2014). Given its role in the health insurance market, lawmakers included two main mechanisms to preserve employer-sponsored health insurance coverage, as well as potentially increase it—an individual mandate and an employer penalty or a "free-rider" penalty.

However, the requirements for employers of a certain size to provide coverage or face "free-rider" penalties—and the methods for calculating the penalties for noncompliant employers—have been administratively complex and fraught with controversy. Throughout the implementation of the ACA, GOP lawmakers and conservative experts have contended that the law will have negative impacts on the labor market by having a dampening effect on hiring and job creation, and reducing the number of hours individuals work to avoid the "free-rider" penalties (Gitis, 2014; Gonshorowski, 2013). In 2011, top House GOP lawmakers released a report entitled "Obamacare: A Budget-Busting Job-Killing Health Care Law" (Boehner et al., 2011). The release of the report coincided with the introduction of legislation to repeal the ACA in the house— "Repeal the Job-Killing Health Care Law Act." Importantly, one of the main arguments the GOP was using to push for near-complete repeal of the ACA was its labor market impacts. Meanwhile, proponents of the ACA maintained that the law would have positive impacts on the labor market primarily by reducing job lock, making it easier for entrepreneurs to start their own job-creating small businesses, and helping business bottom lines by bending the cost curve in health care over time (Carkk, 2011). Some even argued that repealing the ACA would result in a loss of hundreds of thousands of jobs (Cutler, 2011).

The Great Recession—the worst economic downturn since the Great Depression—began in December 2007 and continued through June 2009 (Center on Budget and Policy Priorities, 2014). Over this time, nearly 9 million jobs were lost, with long-term unemployment (defined as those who were unemployed for 27 weeks or more) hitting its highest level in 60 years (Center on Budget and Policy Priorities, 2014). When President Obama took office in January 2009, the economic downturn had slowed, but there was growing concern across the country about the depth and duration of the recession—and questions about what could turn the economy around. In this context, one of the main questions plaguing the ACA was how it would impact the labor market.

The ACA sought to increase the number of people with health insurance in the United States by enacting policies that supported a goal of "shared responsibility." For the nearly 50 million individuals who were uninsured, the law aimed to extend coverage by providing tax credits or premium subsidies for individuals and families with incomes up to 400 percent of the FPL, and by enacting an individual mandate that requires all individuals with access to affordable insurance to purchase it or pay a penalty (DeNavas-Walt, Proctor, and Smith, 2011). The shared responsibility concept also extended to employers—who covered 149 million individuals—or approximately 50 percent of the population (Henry J. Kaiser Family Foundation and Heath Research &Education Trust, 2014). To prevent employers from dropping coverage altogether, the ACA included employer penalties—also known as "free-rider" penalties—that applied to firms with 50 or more full-time workers. However, the methods for calculating full-time workers and the penalties proved to be complicated—and controversial.

Employers with 50 or more full-time workers that did not offer coverage to their employees, or had at least one full-time employee who received a premium tax credit for purchasing coverage through the exchanges would pay $2,000 penalty per full-time employee (exempting the first 30 employees from the penalty). Employers with 50 or more full-time workers that did offer coverage, but that had at least one employee receive a tax credit, would have to pass the lesser of $3,000 for each employee receiving a tax credit or $2,000 for each full-time employee (again exempting the first 30 employees from the penalty). These coverage requirements and penalties were set to go into effect on January 1, 2014, when the coverage expansion started.

One of the most controversial points was defining full-time workers at 30 hours per week to determine which employers would be subject to the penalty. Critics contended that defining full-time employment as 30 hours (instead of following the conventional 40-hour work week) could lead to employers reducing work hours and lower earnings as well (Gitis, 2014). There was also evidence from the Federal Reserve Board that uncertainty on the implementation of the ACA and fiscal policy more generally was making employers "cautious" about hiring new workers and expanding payroll (Federal Reserve Board, 2013). Experts also projected that the 30-hour work week would impact employee behavior by reducing incentives to work by providing subsidies for health insurance to those working below the full-time threshold (Mulligan, 2014).

However, a closer look at the evidence suggests that the ACA has not led to large-scale changes in employment but that some negative labor market impacts have occurred in specific sectors. Industries with low-wage workers and/or those with average work hours near 30 were likely to be most at risk for having their hours reduced to below 30 so that employers were not faced with a free-rider penalty. An analysis by the UC Berkley Labor Center found that the industries with the workers at greatest risk of work hour reduction were restaurants, accommodations, building services, nursing homes, and retail, with restaurant workers being the largest group (Jacobs and Graham-Squire, 2013). However, the analysis found that those at highest risk for work hour reduction accounted for a relatively small percentage of the overall labor force—2.3 million workers or 1.8 percent of the total labor force (Jacobs and Graham-Squire, 2013). Media reports support the conclusion that individual retailers and fast-food chains were reducing work hours for some employees to just below the 30-hour threshold to allow them to either drop insurance or avoid paying the free-rider penalty (Cohn, 2013; Heritage Foundation, 2013).

Generally, widespread reductions in work hours outside of these industries have not been observed. An analysis by the Center on Budget and Policy Priorities examined a number of data sources and concluded that there has not been a significant shift to part-time work following the passage of the ACA (Van de Water, 2015). While there is some evidence that the ACA has spurred employers to shift employees into part-time work, the trend is limited to certain sectors at this time (Figure 4.1).

In addition to the 30-hour threshold for defining full-time workers, there have been reports that exempting businesses with fewer than 50 full-time workers from the employer penalties has had labor market impacts as well. One survey found that employers with fewer than 50 full-time workers were "generally" making more decisions on hiring, reductions, and allocation of work hours (International Foundation of Employee Benefit Plans, 2013). In particular, there were a number of news reports detailing work hour reductions or decisions not to hire in the restaurant industry (Rovner, 2013). However, many of these were anecdotal reports. On the other end of the spectrum, the White House released an analysis in 2013 citing that restaurants had the most rapid growth in employment in the retail and food industry since 2010 (Vandivier, 2013). The analysis also found that from 2009 to 2019, 87 percent of the increase in employment could be attributed to full-time jobs (Vandivier, 2013). Gauging the impact of the ACA on small businesses' hiring practices is hard to quantify. While there is evidence that the ACA has impacted hiring or expansion decisions, overall job growth has been increasing since the passage of the law as the economy generally begins to recover.

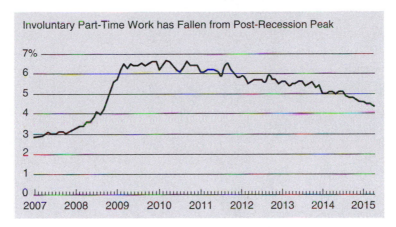

Figure 4.1 Involuntary Part-Time Workers as a Share of All Workers

Note: Figure shows those working part-time for economic reasons, which comprises those working part-time because of slack work or business conditions and those who could only find part-time work.

Source: Van de Water, P. 2015. "Health Reform Not Causing Significant Shift to Part-Time Work but Raising Threshold to 40 Hours a Week Would Make a Sizeable Shift Likely." Center on Budget and Policy Priorities. Accessed January 24, 2015. http://www.cbpp.org/research/health-reform-not-causing-significant-shift-to-part-time-work.

Meanwhile, supporters of the ACA contended that repealing the ACA would reduce the number of jobs in the United States. One analysis projected that if H.R.2, Repealing the Job-Killing Health Care Law Act, were passed, 250,000 to 400,000 jobs would be lost annually (Cutler, 2011). The analysis examined the impacts of potentially higher health care costs if the ACA were to be repealed—which would partially fall on employers and limit their ability to retain or hire more workers (Cutler, 2011). CBO has also weighed in on the ACA's labor market impacts. In 2014, the agency projected that the ACA would reduce work hours by 1.5 to 2 percent from 2017 to 2024—mostly due to individuals choosing to work less (Congressional Budget Office, 2014). However, as others concluded, work hour reductions due to new taxes and the availability of health insurance subsidies would be most concentrated in low-wage workers; therefore, the overall impact on the economy is relatively small (Congressional Budget Office, 2014).

The free-rider penalty and whether it would lead to loss of jobs or shore up employer-sponsored insurance continues to be debated. However, due to technical complexities and political opposition, the Obama

Administration delayed the employer requirements (and penalties in essence) until 2015. The labor market impacts of the ACA—and its 30-hour work week—are yet to be truly measured. Early evidence suggests that low-wage workers in specific industries have seen some declines in hours worked—but widespread job loss due to the ACA has not been observed.

FURTHER READING

Boehner, J., Cantor, E., Camp, D., Kline, J., Ryan, P., and Upton. F. 2011. "Obamacare: A Budget-Busting Job-Killing Health Care Law." Accessed January 3, 2015. http://www.speaker.gov/sites/speaker.house .gov/files/UploadedFiles/ObamaCareReport.pdf.

Carkk, T. 2011. "The Anniversary of the Affordable Care Act: A Year Later the False Attacks Continue." Center for American Progress. January 3, 2015. http://cdn.americanprogress.org/wp-content/uploads/ issues/2011/03/pdf/aca_anniversary.pdf.

Center on Budget and Policy Priorities. 2014. "Chartbook: The Legacy of the Great Recession." Accessed January 5, 2015. http://www.cbpp.org/ cms/index.cfm?fa=view&id=3252.

Centers for Medicare and Medicaid Services. 2014. "Table 1. National Health Expenditures; Aggregate and Per Capita Amounts, Annual Percent Change and Percent Distribution: Selected Calendar Years 1960–2012." Accessed January 3, 2015. http://www.cms.gov/ Research-Statistics-Data-and-Systems/Statistics-Trends-and-Reports/ NationalHealthExpendData/Downloads/Proj2012.pdf.

Cohn, A. 2013. "Obamacare Is Coming: Forever 21 Slashes Workers' Hours." Daily Signal. Accessed January 6, 2015. http://dailysignal.com/ 2013/08/19/obamacare-is-coming-forever-21-slashes-workers-hours/.

Congressional Budget Office. 2014. "Labor Market Effects of the Afford-able Care Act: Updated Estimates. The Budget and Economic Out-look: 2014 to 2024." Accessed January 6, 2015. http://www.cbo.gov/ sites/default/files/cbofiles/attachments/45010-breakout-AppendixC .pdf.

Cutler, D. 2011. "Repealing ACA Is a Job-Killer." Center for American Progress. Accessed January 3, 2015. https://www.americanprogress.org/ issues/healthcare/report/2011/01/07/8887/repealing-health-care- is-a-job-killer/.

DeNavas-Walt, C., Proctor, B., and Smith, J. 2011. "Income, Poverty, and Health Insurance Coverage in the United States: 2010." U.S. Cen-sus Bureau. Accessed January 5, 2015. https://www.census.gov/prod/ 2011pubs/p60-239.pdf.

Federal Reserve Board. 2013. "Summary of Commentary on Current Economic Conditions by Federal Reserve District. Beige Book—October 16,
2013." Accessed January 6, 2015. http://www.federalreserve.gov/mone
tarypolicy/beigebook/beigebook201310.htm.

Gitis, B. 2014. "The Problem with ACA's 30 Hour Work Week." American Action Forum. Accessed January 3, 2014. http://americanactionfo
rum.org/insights/the-problem-with-acas-30-hour-work-week.

Gonshorowski, D. 2013. "The Affordable Care Act Negatively Impacts the
Labor Supply." Heritage Foundation. Accessed January 3, 2015. http://
www.heritage.org/research/reports/2013/03/impact-of-the-patient-
protection-and-affordable-care-act-on-labor-supply.

Henry J. Kaiser Family Foundation and Health Research & Educational Trust. 2014. "Employer Health Benefits: 2014 Annual Survey."
Accessed January 3, 2015. http://files.kff.org/attachment/2014-employer-
health-benefits-survey-full-report.

H.R.2. 2011. "Repeal the Job-Killing Health Care Law Act." Accessed
January 3, 2015. https://www.govtrack.us/congress/bills/112/hr2.

Heritage Foundation. 2013. "Obamacare Threatens Fast Food Workers with
Reduced Hours." Accessed January 6, 2015. http://obamacare.heritage.org/
obamacare-threatens-fast-food-workers-nationwide-with-reduced-hours/.

International Foundation of Employee Benefit Plans. 2013. "2013 Employer
Sponsored Health Care: ACA's Impact." Accessed January 10, 2015.
http://www.ifebp.org/pdf/research/2103ACAImpactSurvey.pdf.

Jacobs, K. and Graham-Squire, D. 2013. Under the "Forty Hours is Full
Time Act" More Americans Would Lose Job-Based Health Coverage and Work Hours, While Federal Costs Would Increase. UC Berkley
Labor Center. Accessed October 6, 2015. http://laborcenter.berkeley
.edu/under-the-forty-hours-is-full-time-act-more-american-would-
lose-job-based-health-coverage-and-work-hours-while-federal-costs-
would-increase/.

Mulligan, C. 2014. "The Affordable Care Act and the New Economics of Part-Time Work." Mercatus Center, George Mason University.
Accessed January 6, 2015. http://mercatus.org/publication/affordable-
care-act-and-new-economics-part-time-work.

Payne, A. 2013. "How Obamacare Hurts If You're Looking for a Job." Daily
Signal. Accessed January 6, 2015. http://dailysignal.com/2013/10/23/
how-obamacare-hurts-you-if-youre-looking-for-a-job/.

Rovner, J. 2013. "Will Obamacare Mean Fewer Jobs? Depends on Whom
You Ask." National Public Radio. Accessed January 10, 2015. http://
www.npr.org/blogs/health/2013/07/30/207043184/Definition-Of-Full-
Time-A-Sticking-Point-In-Obamacare.

Van de Water, P. 2015. "Health Reform Not Causing Significant Shift to Part-Time Work but Raising Threshold to 40 Hours a Week Would Make a Sizeable Shift Likely." Center on Budget and Policy Priorities. Accessed January 24, 2015. http://www.cbpp.org/research/health-reform-not-causing-significant-shift-to-part-time-work.

Vandivier, D. 2013. "What the Affordable Care Act Really Means for Job Growth." White House. Accessed January 10, 2015. http://www.white house.gov/blog/2013/07/29/what-affordable-care-act-really-means-job.

Q21. HAS THE AFFORDABLE CARE ACT INCREASED HEALTH CARE COSTS FOR BUSINESSES?

Answer: The ACA has had both positive and negative impacts on large and small businesses. The main goals of the ACA were to sustainably expand coverage to the uninsured and to slow the growth in health care spending for public and private payers. For small businesses in particular, the law included provisions to make coverage more affordable over the long term. In addition, a wide range of payment and delivery reforms aimed to bend the cost curve in health care - theoretically benefiting all purchasers of health care coverage including employers. However, there are a number of new insurance market requirements on both small and large businesses that make the impacts on employers more complicated. Disentangling the net effect of these different provisions is a complex undertaking, and both supporters and opponents of Obamacare have sometimes cherry-picked this data to support their positions.

The Facts: While the Administration and supporters of the ACA contend that the law has helped businesses—especially small businesses—opponents believe it has increased costs and limited job growth. Historically, small businesses have faced volatile premium prices from one year to the next and limited coverage options, among other issues. The ACA sought to address these issues by creating a health insurance exchange for small businesses—the Small Business Health Options Program (SHOP)—and by providing tax credits to offset the cost of coverage.

The Democratic Policy Committee and the Senate Finance Committee among others all released briefs and fact sheets detailing the ways the law would help small businesses (Democratic Policy Committee, 2010; Senate Finance Committee, 2010; The White House, 2014). The ACA also included a number of payment and delivery reforms that were intended to slow health care cost growth for all employers—including large employers.

The law also placed new requirements on businesses to comply with insurance market reforms, such as requiring that all plans sold on the small-group market cover the EHB package. Compliance with the market reforms has required businesses to purchase more comprehensive coverage in many cases and increased administrative burdens to ensure compliance with the law. As a result, opponents of the law have cited that the new market reforms, as well as new taxes in the ACA, increased costs to all businesses (Senger, 2014). One analysis went so far as to project that the ACA will increase costs to large businesses by an additional 8 percent by 2023 (Troy and Wilson, 2014). While the impact of the ACA on small and large businesses will take years to unfold, the tax credits and the SHOP exchange have not been successful in the early years—and most businesses have initially faced increased costs at least partially attributable to the ACA.

Small businesses have been subject to increasing costs and volatile premium prices—leading to fewer small businesses offering coverage over the past several years. For instance, small businesses (defined as those with fewer than 200 workers) have seen premiums increase 63 percent from 2004 through 2014, and since 1999, the percentage of small businesses providing coverage has steadily decreased from 65 percent to 54 percent (Henry J. Kaiser Family Foundation and Heath Research & Education Trust, 2014). As a result of these cost pressures, small businesses are less likely to offer coverage to employees than large businesses. An estimated 54 percent of small businesses offer health coverage compared to 98 percent of large firms (those with 200 or more employees; Henry J. Kaiser Family Foundation and Heath Research & Education Trust, 2014).

In response to these trends, the ACA established a tax credit program that began in 2010 to defray the cost of coverage for employers with fewer than 25 workers, and to offer an incentive for employers not offering coverage to do so. However, a small percentage of eligible businesses have utilized the tax credit. The Government Accountability Office (GAO) studied how often the tax credit is claimed, factors that limit participation in the program, and data needed to assess the effects of the tax credit program, among other issues (Government Accountability Office, 2012). The GAO found that in 2010 only 170,000 out of 1.4 to 4 million potentially eligible businesses claimed the credit (Government Accountability Office, 2012). One of the main flaws of this policy proposal is that the majority of employers with fewer than 25 employees—83 percent—do not offer health insurance to begin with (Government Accountability Office, 2012). While the tax credit defrayed the cost of providing coverage for a minority of eligible businesses, it did not incent businesses that are not offering coverage to start.

The ACA also established the SHOP exchanges for businesses with up to 100 workers. In the SHOP exchanges, small business employees can purchase plans that comply with the new ACA insurance market reforms and coverage requirements. To maintain small employer coverage—and to perhaps even increase it—the SHOP exchanges aimed to create predictable eligibility and participation requirements, to spur competition among plans to constrain (or stabilize) premium growth, to increase plan choice while allowing employers to make predictable contributions toward the cost of coverage, and to create a convenient online portal for plan selection (Dash, Lucia, and Thomas, 2014). However, the SHOP exchanges have experienced a rocky start. Some SHOP exchanges run by states were not ready to enroll individuals on January 1, 2014, and the Federal SHOP exchange, which served 33 states, delayed important features of the exchange such as online enrollment and employee choice of plans (Dash, Lucia, and Thomas, 2014). As a result, evaluating their long-term impact on premium volatility and affordability of coverage for small businesses is difficult.

At the same time that the ACA included these new benefits for small businesses, a number of new requirements were placed on both small and large businesses. First, the small-group market became subject to new insurance market reforms that largely went into effect in 2014. For instance, small-group plans must adhere to new premium rating and variation requirements, provide the EHB package, and cannot deny coverage based on preexisting conditions. Large businesses are required to offer a minimum level of coverage—termed minimum essential coverage—to employees or face a penalty. Large businesses are also subject to new reporting requirements, waiting period requirements for new employees, new taxes on high-cost plans, maintaining young adults on their parents' policies until 26 years of age, requiring coverage with no cost-sharing for approved preventive services, and contributing to the Patient-Centered Outcomes Research Institute.

Taken together, these requirements have led to employers reporting increased costs. In a survey by the Federal Reserve Bank of New York, manufacturing and service firms reported a 9 to 10 percent increase in the costs of coverage—although the increase could not be attributed solely to the ACA (Federal Reserve Bank of New York, 2014). The majority of employers surveyed reported that the ACA increased their costs (Federal Reserve Bank of New York, 2014). Other studies have tried to quantify the impacts of the ACA on large businesses. One survey projected that the ACA would cost large businesses with more than 10,000 employees $4,800 to $5,900 per employee and that their costs would be 8 percent higher by 2023 as a result of the ACA (Troy and Wilson, 2014). However, the analysis did not take into account factors such as the rate of health care inflation, other cost trends forcing employers to make changes to their benefits, or savings from the ACA that could offset some of these costs (Millman, 2014; Troy and Wilson, 2014). While employers are reporting increased costs, quantifying the impact with an agreed-upon methodology has been difficult.

At the same time that employers are reporting increased costs due to the ACA, employer premiums increased an average of only 3 percent from 2013 to 2014 when many of the requirements went into effect (Henry J. Kaiser Family Foundation and Heath Research & Education Trust, 2014). The historically low growth in the cost of employer-sponsored coverage runs counter to the results of employer surveys.

This suggests that the ACA is likely increasing costs to some employers, but that other trends are constraining premium growth—such as new payment and delivery reforms, as well as increasing the share employees pay toward their health care in the form of higher premiums, deductibles, and co-pays. Weighing the impact of the ACA's provisions aimed at assisting employers via the SHOP exchanges and payment and delivery reforms to slow health care cost growth against the new insurance market reform and coverage requirements, as well as new fees, will take several years. However, in the short term at least, the ACA appears to have at least modestly increased costs for many businesses.

FURTHER READING

Dash, S., Lucia, K., and Thomas, A. 2014. "Implementing the Affordable Care Act: State Action to Establish SHOP Marketplaces." The Commonwealth Fund. Accessed January 20, 2015. http://www.commonwealthfund.org/~/media/files/publications/issue-brief/2014/mar/1735_dash_implementing_aca_state_action_shop_marketplaces_rb.pdf.

Democratic Policy Committee. 2010. "Ensuring Affordable Choices for Small Businesses." Accessed January 19, 2015. http://www.dpc.senate.gov/dpcissue-sen_health_care_bill.cfm.

Federal Reserve Bank of New York. 2014. "Firms Assess Effects of Affordable Care Act." Accessed January 20, 2015. http://www.newyorkfed.org/survey/business_leaders/2014/2014_08Supplemental.pdf.

Government Accountability Office. 2012. "Small Employer Tax Credit: Factors Contributing to Low Use and Complexity." Accessed January 19, 2015. http://gao.gov/assets/600/590832.pdf.

Henry J. Kaiser Family Foundation and Health Research Educational Trust. 2014. "Employer Health Benefits: 2014 Annual Survey." Accessed January 3, 2015. http://files.kff.org/attachment/2014-employer-health-benefits-survey-full-report.

Millman, J. 2014. "Large Employers See Costs from Obamacare." *The Washington Post.* Accessed January 20, 2015. http://www.washingtonpost.com/blogs/wonkblog/wp/2014/04/01/large-employers-see-costs-from-obamacare/.

Senate Finance Committee. 2010. "Affordable Care for Small Businesses: Increasing Choice, Protecting Workers." Accessed January 19, 2015. http://www.finance.senate.gov/newsroom/chairman/release/?id=6384 077c-4de8-421a-8ac7-b0fc5a2e8847.

Senger, A. 2014. "3 Things Obamacare Is Doing to Workplace Health Coverage." *The Daily Signal.* Accessed January 19, 2015. http://dailysignal .com/2014/05/21/3-things-obamacare-workplace-health-coverage/.

Troy, T., and Wilson, D. 2014. "The Cost of the Affordable Care Act to Large Employers." American Health Policy Institute. Accessed January 19, 2015. http://www.americanhealthpolicy.org/content/documents/resour ces/2014_ACA_Cost_Study.pdf.

The White House. 2014. "Health Reform for Small Businesses: The Affordable Care Act Increases Choice and Saving Money for Small Businesses." Accessed January 19, 2015. http://www.whitehouse.gov/ files/documents/health_reform_for_small_businesses.pdf.

Q22. DOES THE AFFORDABLE CARE ACT ACTUALLY HELP SMALL BUSINESSES BY REDUCING ADMINISTRATIVE COSTS AND PREMIUM VOLATILITY?

Answer: Unknown at this point. There are some indications that ACA requirements may be a contributing factor in rising health care administrative costs, but defenders of Obamacare note that its provisions may be playing an important role in reducing premium volatility and inflation, which has historically been a major problem for employers.

The Facts: The ACA reformed two major insurance markets—the individual- and small-group markets. The latter serves small businesses, which the ACA defines as firms with 100 employees or less (National Association of Insurance Commissioners, 2010).

The ACA set out to reform both the individual- and small-group markets. While some of the problems in each market are distinct, both individuals and small businesses were often subject to sharp increases in premiums from one year to the next. On average, from 1999 to 2014 small business premiums (for firms with fewer than 200 employees) increased by 7 percent—although in some years increases were as high as nearly 15 percent (Henry J. Kaiser Family Foundation and Health Research & Education Trust, 2014). Increasing premiums often led to small businesses dropping coverage. The same survey reported that in 1999 65 percent of small businesses with fewer than 200 workers offered coverage, but this number dropped to 54 percent by 2014 (Henry J. Kaiser Family Foundation and Health Research & Education Trust, 2014).

In response, the ACA sought to stabilize premiums, as well as stem the erosion of coverage, in the small-group market primarily by establishing SHOP exchanges. The SHOP exchanges were intended to reduce administrative costs for small businesses through a convenient, online shopping portal for employees, and to make premiums more stable by pooling risk across small businesses. The SHOP exchanges are only open to small businesses initially, which the ACA defines as firms with 1 to 100 employees; however, until 2016 the law gives states the option to define the small-group market as firms with up to 50 employees and starting in 2017 states have the option to allow large businesses to use the exchanges as well (National Association of Insurance Commissioners, 2010).

Like the individual market reforms, the SHOP exchanges were set to launch in 2014 at the same time that small businesses were subject to new rating rules. One critical market reform to try to stabilize rates across businesses prohibited insurers from varying premiums based on health status. In essence, this would increase rates for businesses with younger and healthier workers and decrease costs for firms with older and sicker workers. Over time, premium increases could theoretically be stabilized, but rate increases were most likely to be acute in 2014 when the market reforms went into effect. The Centers for Medicare and Medicaid Services Office of the Actuary (OACT) estimated that 65 percent of small businesses offering coverage would experience an increase in rates due to the new ACA rating rules because their premiums were below the average (Centers for Medicare and Medicaid Services Office of the Actuary, 2014). The OACT study fueled the political controversy over the impacts of the ACA on small businesses. Speaker Boehner released the following statement in response to the report:

> The Obama administration has finally been forced to disclose what we've long feared: the president's health care law means higher premiums for millions of American workers. For all the promises

of lower costs for small businesses, the administration now admits that far more of these workers will pay higher than lower premiums under the law. This broken promise comes in the form of lower take-home pay for some of the hardest-working people in this country. Two-thirds of these Americans—11 million people—will see more money coming out of their paycheck every month, according to the president's own actuaries. . . . Two-thirds of small business employers face higher premiums as well, which is one of the reasons so many are struggling to create jobs under the president's law. (Boehner, 2014)

Over time variation in premiums across employers and individuals should be minimized as a result of the ACA because of prohibition on rating-based health status and the pooling of risk across businesses (Blumberg and Holahan, 2014). However, OACT's analysis suggested that in 2014, a majority of small businesses across the country would experience rate hikes that are at least partially attributable to the ACA (Centers for Medicare and Medicaid Services Office of the Actuary, 2014).

However, small businesses were seeing some of the lowest premium increases over the past 15 years. From 2013 to 2014, the Henry J. Kaiser Family Foundation reported that average small family premiums increased by 1.7 percent (Henry J. Kaiser Family Foundation and Health Research & Education Trust, 2014). This was the lowest increase since the survey began in 1999, suggesting that other economic and policy trends could be constraining cost growth. Since 2000, the average annual increase was 5.5 percent and there were at least three years where double-digit increases were observed (Blumberg and Holahan, 2014; Henry J. Kaiser Family Foundation and Health Research Education Trust, 2014). Given these historical cost trends, coupled with the new market reforms in the ACA, increases would be expected to be higher on average than observed in 2014.

The true impacts of the ACA on small businesses cannot be assessed until the SHOP exchanges are fully functional. In the meantime, most small businesses have been experiencing significant premium cost growth over the last decade and a half. There is evidence that the ACA increased costs for a majority of businesses due to its insurance market reforms; however, at the same time, other factors—some of them at least partially attributable to Obamacare—appear to be slowing health care cost growth generally. For instance, the Medicare payment reductions and value-based payment reforms in the ACA are placing new pressures on payers and providers to become more efficient and cannot be ruled out as contributing to the slower cost growth in health care generally, and employers are increasingly offering benefit designs shift costs to employees via higher deductibles and cost-sharing. These and other factors could be moderating cost growth in the small business market (even as new market reforms increase premiums for some businesses) as evidenced by the lowest increase in small business premiums in 2014 than in the past 15 years.

FURTHER READING

Blumberg, L., and Holahan, J. 2014. "Year-to-Year Variation in Small-Group Health Insurance Premiums: Double-Digit Annual Increases Have Been Common over the Past Decade." Urban Institute. Accessed January 23, 2015. http://www.rwjf.org/content/dam/farm/reports/issue_briefs/2014/rwjf415555.

Boehner, J. 2014. "Obama Admin: Two Thirds of Small Businesses to See Premiums Spike under Obamacare." Accessed May 22, 2015. http://www.speaker.gov/press-release/obama-administration-two-thirds-small-businesses-see-premiums-spike-under-obamacare.

Centers for Medicare and Medicaid Services Office of the Actuary. 2014. "Report to Congress on the Impact on Premiums for Individuals and Families with Employer-Sponsored Health Insurance from the Guaranteed Issue, Guaranteed Renewal, and Fair Health Insurance Premiums Provisions of the Affordable Care Act." Accessed January 22, 2015. https://www.cms.gov/Research-Statistics-Data-and-Systems/Research/ActuarialStudies/Downloads/ACA-Employer-Premium-Impact.pdf.

Gitis, B., Ryan, C., and Batkins, S. 2014. "Obamacare's Impact on Small Business Wages and Employment." American Action Forum. Accessed January 22, 2015. http://americanactionforum.org/research/obamacares-impact-on-small-business-wages-and-employment.

Henry J. Kaiser Family Foundation and Health Research Educational Trust. 2014. "Employer Health Benefits: 2014 Annual Survey." Accessed January 3, 2015. http://files.kff.org/attachment/2014-employer-health-benefits-survey-full-report.

Matusiak, A. 2013. "Five Ways the Affordable Care Act Helps America's Small Businesses." *The White House Blog.* Accessed January 22, 2015. http://www.whitehouse.gov/blog/2013/08/14/five-ways-affordable-care-act-helps-america-s-small-businesses.

National Association of Insurance Commissioners. 2010. "Patient Protection and Affordable Care Act of 2009: Health Insurance Exchanges." Accessed October 6, 2015. http://www.naic.org/documents/committees_b_Exchanges.pdf.

Senate Finance Committee. 2009. "Affordable Care for Small Businesses: Increasing Choice, Protecting Workers." Accessed January 22, 2015. http://www.finance.senate.gov/newsroom/chairman/release/?id=63840 77c-4de8-421a-8ac7-b0fc5a2e8847.

The White House, Office of the Press Secretary. 2009. "Remarks by the President to a Joint Session of Congress on Health Care." Accessed January 22, 2015. http://www.whitehouse.gov/the_press_office/Remarks-by-the-President-to-a-Joint-Session-of-Congress-on-Health-Care.

Q23. ARE EMPLOYERS CHANGING OR LIMITING THE HEALTH COVERAGE OPTIONS THEY PROVIDE TO EMPLOYEES IN RESPONSE TO THE AFFORDABLE CARE ACT?

Answer: Yes, but many of these changes were anticipated—even desired—by the architects of the ACA. The ACA includes numerous changes that impact both large and small employers. The changes include new requirements on whom employer-sponsored health plans must cover and what they must cover in terms of services and cost-sharing, as well as new taxes on insurance policies. The requirement and changes are being implemented over several years—from 2010 to 2018.

The Facts: Employer health plans are subject to a host of new requirements under the ACA. The changes began soon after the law passed in 2010 and continue to be enacted through 2018. They range from changes in whom employers must cover and to what they must cover, as well as new penalties and taxes on high-cost insurance plans. The breadth of changes affecting both large and small employers has required many to make changes to the health plans they offer—and begin to think about future changes in benefits in response to ACA provisions that have not yet gone into effect.

The Administration emphasized on repeated occasions that individuals who like their plans would be able to keep them (Jacobson, 2013). Meanwhile, opponents of the ACA have emphasized that the law would change employer benefits in response to direct requirements on employers plans, as well as indirect effects from increased costs (Senger, 2014). Surveys of large employers (those with 1,000 employees or more) indicate that the vast majority—95 percent—believe that providing health care coverage for employees will be a critical part of their benefits package (Towers Watson, 2014). At the same time, 94 percent of employers surveyed also stated that they anticipate employer-sponsored insurance will undergo modest or major changes (Towers Watson, 2014). While the ACA has not led to a significant erosion in employer-sponsored insurance, it has changed the coverage itself for many Americans and will continue to do so as the employer requirements take full effect.

First, the ACA required that employers must allow children up to age 26 years to remain on their parents' plans starting in 2010. The reasons for this policy are threefold: (1) young adults previously had the highest rate of uninsurance of any age group, (2) young adults are the least likely to have access to employer-sponsored health insurance, and (3) an estimated one out of six young adults has a chronic illness (Centers for Medicare and Medicaid Services, 2014). In the first year after the policy was enacted, an estimated 2.5 million young adults were estimated to gain coverage (Sommers and Schwartz, 2011).

The ACA also included a number of coverage requirements that affected small and large employers. First, the ACA requires that all individuals be enrolled in "minimum essential coverage" to comply with the individual mandate, which employer-sponsored insurance can fulfill. While most employer plans meet minimum essential coverage requirements, there are a minority of employers that have likely had to come into compliance with this requirement. Second, employers are required to provide health plans that meet minimum value requirements, which are defined as having at least a 60 percent actuarial value. Actuarial value is defined as the average proportion of medical expenses an insurer pays for a standard population. Therefore, a 60 percent actuarial value would mean that on average, the insurer would be expected to pay 60 percent of the medical costs incurred and the individual or family would pay 40 percent on average. The vast majority of large and small and employer plans have an actuarial value of at least 60 percent—an estimated 1.6 to 2 percent of employer plans did not as of 2012 and likely had to change their plans to meet this requirement (Grassli and Klinger, 2014). In addition, small-group plans are required to comply with the EHB package and its 10 covered categories. While large employer plans do not have to comply with the EHB, most large employers include benefits with a scope similar to the ACA EHB categories (Grassli and Klinger, 2014). However, they have had to comply with other reforms such as the prohibition on annual or lifetime limits on EHB categories, which likely required changes in plan design to come into compliance.

Another example of coverage changes employers had to make after the ACA was offering plans that covered certain preventive services with zero dollar cost-sharing for enrollees. The ACA requires that preventive services with an "A" or "B" rating from the United States Preventive Services Task Force, immunizations that are routinely used and recommended by the Advisory Committee on Immunization Practices, and other screenings recommended for women and children by the Health Resources and Services Administration not be subject to cost-sharing. For instance, this would include services such as breast cancer or colorectal cancer screenings. As a result of this new coverage policy, 41 percent of workers covered by employer-sponsored health plans saw changes in the preventive services covered, and 33 experienced changed cost-sharing (Henry J. Kaiser Family Foundation and Health Research & Educational Trust, 2012). In total, the Assistance Secretary for Planning and Evaluation estimated that 76 million individuals gained access to preventive services (Burke and Simmons, 2014). Over time, this policy will likely mean that few individuals with commercial insurance will experience financial barriers to receiving preventive care (Henry J. Kaiser Family Foundation, 2014). However, it is clear that both large- and small-group employers had to modify their plans to comply with this new requirement.

Last, the high-cost plan excise tax—or the "Cadillac tax"—is another controversial employer-related provision. Currently, employer contributions toward health insurance are not treated like wages—these contributions are exempt from income and payroll taxes. In addition, employee contributions to coverage are usually exempt from income and payroll taxes. CBO stated:

> The favorable tax treatment of employment-based health insurance is the largest single tax expenditure by the federal government. (Tax expenditures are exclusions, deductions, preferential rates, and credits in the tax system that resemble federal spending by providing financial assistance to specific activities, entities, or groups of people.) Excluding employment-based health insurance from both income and payroll taxes will cost the government $248 billion in 2013. (Congressional Budget Office, 2013)

As a result, economists project, the tax benefit makes enrollees in these generous plans more likely to overutilize services because they are subject to little or no cost-sharing and also favors those with higher incomes because they have higher income tax rates and benefit more from the tax exclusion (Piotrowski, 2013). The excise tax is designed to reduce the generosity of employer-sponsored benefits over time—and help drive down overall health care cost growth.

An earlier version of the health reform legislation had the provision slated to go into effect in 2013; however, it was pushed out to 2018 amid concerns from employers and unions (Egan, 2013). The Cadillac tax imposes an annual 40 percent excise tax on the cost of health insurance coverage above $10,200 for individual coverage and $27,500 for family coverage starting in 2018 (note that the thresholds grow with inflation starting in 2020). In general, the Cadillac tax takes aim at employer-sponsored health plans with generous benefits and low-cost sharing for employees. If employers did not modify their benefits to remain below these thresholds, CBO estimates that in 2018 20 percent of all individuals enrolled in an employer-sponsored health plan would have coverage subject to the tax (Congressional Budget Office, 2013). An estimated 25 percent of employers in one survey reported making changes to their plans in 2014—far in advance of 2018 to ensure the value of their plans does not exceed the thresholds in the law (International Federation of Employer Benefit Plans, 2014). While the goal of the Cadillac tax is to retrain health care cost growth, it will continue to require employers to modify the generosity of their plans to avoid the excise tax.

Taken together, the new coverage requirements for whom employers must cover, what they must cover, and the new taxes have required both small and large businesses to make changes to their health insurance plans. While many changes expanding coverage occurred for the 2014 plan year, limitations in coverage could be on the horizon as the Cadillac tax goes into effect.

FURTHER READING

Burke, A., and Simmons, A. 2014. "Increased Coverage of Preventive Services with Zero Cost-Sharing under the Affordable Care Act." Assistant Secretary for Planning and Evaluation, Department of Health and Human Services. Accessed January 26, 2015. http://aspe.hhs.gov/health/reports/2014/PreventiveServices/ib_PreventiveServices.pdf.

Centers for Medicare and Medicaid Services. 2012. "Patient Protection and Affordable Care Act; Standards Related to Essential Health Benefits, Actuarial Value, and Accreditation." Center for Consumer Information and Insurance Oversight. Accessed January 25, 2015. http://www.gpo.gov/fdsys/pkg/FR-2012-11-26/pdf/2012-28362.pdf.

Centers for Medicare and Medicaid Services. 2014. "Young Adults and the Affordable Care Act: Protecting Young Adults and Eliminating Burdens on Families and Businesses." Center for Consumer Information and Insurance Oversight. Accessed January 24, 2015. http://www.cms.gov/CCIIO/Resources/Files/adult_child_fact_sheet.html.

Congressional Budget Office. 2013. "Options for Reducing the Deficit: 2014 to 2023." Accessed January 26, 2015. http://www.cbo.gov/sites/default/files/cbofiles/attachments/44715-OptionsForReducingDeficit-3.pdf.

Egan, E. 2013. "Primer: Cadillac Tax (High-Cost Plan Excise Tax)." American Action Forum. Accessed January 26, 2015. http://americanaction forum.org/sites/default/files/Cadillac%20Tax%20Primer%20Final.pdf.

Grassli, S., and Klinger, L. 2014. "Understanding the Difference between Minimum Essential Coverage, Essential Health Benefits, Minimum Value, and Actuarial Value." Leavitt Group. Accessed January 25, 2015. https://news.leavitt.com/health-care-reform/understanding-diffe rence-minimum-essential-coverage-essential-health-benefits-mini mum-value-actuarial-value/.

Henry J. Kaiser Family Foundation. 2014. "Preventive Services Covered by Private Health Plans under the Affordable Care Act." Accessed January 26, 2015. http://kff.org/health-reform/fact-sheet/preventive-service s-covered-by-private-health-plans/.

Henry J. Kaiser Family Foundation and Health Research Educational Trust. 2012. "Employer Health Benefits: 2012 Annual Survey." Accessed January 26, 2015. https://kaiserfamilyfoundation.files.wordpress.com/2013/ 03/8345-employer-health-benefits-annual-survey-full-report-0912.pdf.

International Federation of Employer Benefit Plans. 2014. "New International Foundation Survey Finds Majority of Employers Believe ACA Has Had Negative Impact on Their Company." Accessed January 26, 2015. https://www.ifebp.org/aboutus/pressroom/releases/Pages/ pr_061114.aspx.

Jacobson, L. 2013. "Barack Obama Says That What He'd Said Was You Could Keep Your Plan 'If It Hasn't Changed since the Law Passed.'" Accessed November 6, 2014. http://www.politifact.com/truth-o-meter/ statements/2013/nov/06/barack-obama/barack-obama-says-what-hed- said-was-you-could-keep/.

Piotrowski, J. 2013. "Excise Tax on 'Cadillac' Plans." *Health Affairs*. Health Policy Briefs. Accessed January 26, 2015. http://www.healthaf fairs.org/healthpolicybriefs/brief.php?brief_id=99.

Senger, A. 2014. "3 Things Obamacare Is Doing to Workplace Health Coverage." *The Daily Signal*. Accessed January 19, 2015. http://dailysig nal.com/2014/05/21/3-things-obamacare-workplace-health-coverage/.

Sommers, B., and Schwartz, K. 2011. "2.5 Million Young Adults Gain Health Insurance Due to the Affordable Care Act." Department of Health and Human Services, Assistant Secretary for Planning and Evaluation. Accessed January 24, 2015. http://www.aspe.hhs.gov/ health/reports/2011/YoungAdultsACA/ib.pdf.

Towers Watson. 2014. "Executive Summary: Towers Watson/NBGH Employer Survey on Purchasing Value in Health Care." Accessed January 24, 2015. http://www.towerswatson.com/en-US/Insights/IC-Types/Survey-Research-Results/2014/03/towers-watson-nbgh-employer-survey-on-purchasing-value-in-health-care/.

UPS. 2013. "Working Spouse Eligibility: Frequently Asked Questions." Accessed January 24, 2015. https://kaiserhealthnews.files.wordpress.com/2013/08/ups-spousal-coverage.pdf.

Q24. DOES THE AFFORDABLE CARE ACT REDUCE "JOB LOCK" AND PROMOTE ENTREPRENEURSHIP?

Answer: In theory, yes, because it provides Americans with additional flexibility in health insurance options outside of the traditional employer-based system. But while anecdotal evidence suggests that some Americans are taking advantage of the ACA to leave employers and launch their own business ventures, the exact impact is difficult to quantify at this early juncture in the ACA's implementation.

The Facts: Job lock is defined as workers not being able to switch jobs or start their own businesses because of the need to maintain employer-sponsored insurance. Supporters of the ACA cite a reduction in job lock as an additional benefit of the law's insurance exchanges and subsidies. For instance, the White House released multiple statements and blog posts during and after the health reform debate, stating that the law would eventually reduce job lock (Chopra, 2009; Furman, 2014; Romer, 2009). The idea is that the availability of insurance for those with pre-existing conditions or need for health insurance through exchanges (and new premium subsidies for qualifying individuals) would allow people formerly tied to their jobs for health insurance to become entrepreneurs or take jobs at small firms that may not provide insurance.

Meanwhile, opponents of the ACA have focused more on alleged negative labor market impacts resulting from the law, such as reduction in work hours and employer caution in hiring (Gitis, 2014; Gonshorowski, 2013). Unfortunately, job lock is difficult to study. While there have been some early efforts to assess the ACA's impact on job lock and promoting entrepreneurship, in general research on the topic has not been robust.

Labor economics indicates that when workers have the option to change jobs or enter or exit the labor market, they are likely to take jobs where they can be most productive (Government Accountability Office, 2011). This resulting job mobility is theorized to create labor market efficiencies and benefit the broader economy (Government Accountability Office, 2011). While a number of factors impact job mobility such as wages and employment options, one of the most relevant factors in health care has been the benefit of employer-sponsored insurance. Job lock in the context of health care refers to workers remaining in jobs that they would otherwise leave because of the risk of losing health coverage or continuity in health care providers due to a lack of portability of coverage across jobs (Fairlie, Kapur, and Gates, 2010; Government Accountability Office, 2011). The impacts of job lock are largely regarded negatively because they impede individuals' choices to start their own businesses, work for start-ups or small businesses, work fewer hours, or leave the workforce temporarily (or permanently) for personal reasons (Government Accountability Office, 2011).

Approximately 50 percent of Americans or an estimated 149 million individuals below the age of 65 have employer-sponsored health insurance (Henry J. Kaiser Family Foundation and Health Research & Educational Trust, 2014). Given the numbers of Americans reliant on employers for coverage, both Democrats and Republicans have believed that health insurance–related job lock has impeded job mobility and entrepreneurship. During the 2008 Presidential elections, Republican nominee Sen. John McCain's health care plan would have changed the tax treatment of employer-sponsored health insurance to promote portability of coverage across jobs (Moffit and Owcharkenko, 2008). Representative Paul Ryan (R-WI) and former 2012 Republican Vice Presidential Nominee also released a health reform bill with other Republicans members of Congress that included measures to reduce job lock and allow individuals to take their health insurance benefits with them when they change employment (H.R. 2520, 2009).

During the health reform debate, senior White House economist Christine Romer cited that a benefit of health reform would be to increase entrepreneurship and job productivity (Romer, 2009). Former Chief Technology Officer, Aneesh Chopra reported that after meeting with business leaders all over the country, he often heard the message that the high cost of health insurance was also inhibiting job growth (Chopra, 2009). One of the hopes supporters of health reform repeatedly expressed was that by providing affordable health insurance options for individuals outside of the employer market, job mobility would increase, with more individuals choosing to start their own businesses, work for small firms that could not afford to provide coverage, or have the flexibility to exit the workforce temporarily or permanently for personal reasons such as caring for children or retirement.

While the phenomenon of job lock makes sense intuitively, it is not easy to assess. A 2010 RAND study aimed to address the lack of research on the issue. The study found measurable effects of job lock due to employer-sponsored insurance, which in effect discouraged entrepreneurship (Fairlie, Kapur, and Gates, 2010). For instance, among low-wage workers, those with employer health coverage through a spouse were more likely to start their own businesses than those that did not (Fairlie, Kapur, and Gates, 2010). A 2011 Government Accountability Office study made a similar conclusion—that some workers are more likely to experience job lock to maintain employer-sponsored insurance (Government Accountability Office, 2011).

Given that assessing job lock in general has been difficult from a research perspective, it is understandably difficult to assess the effects of the ACA on job lock. However, a group of Urban Institute and Georgetown University's Center on Health Insurance Reforms researchers projected the state-by-state impact of the ACA on self-employment (Blumberg, Corlette, and Lucia, 2013). The study projected that due to the ACA's insurance market reforms and premium subsidies to assist with purchasing coverage through the exchanges, an estimated 1.5 million more people would be self-employed—an increase of 11 percent (Blumberg, Corlette, and Lucia, 2013). Another study examined the impact of health reform in Massachusetts on self-employment. Unsurprisingly, the study found that the uninsured rate among self-employed individuals fell after Massachusetts implemented its health reform (Tuzeman and Becker, 2014). More interestingly, the study concluded that health reform in the state promoted self-employment as evidenced by the fact that the self-employment rate before and after health reform remained steady in Massachusetts, while it decreased across the nation and in the Northeast (Tuzeman and Becker, 2014). Thus, there is some evidence that the ACA may promote—or at least maintain—current levels of self-employment.

The Congressional Budget Office has also examined the impacts of the ACA on labor markets, which sparked significant political controversy. A 2014 CBO analysis projected that the ACA would lead to 2 to 2.5 million fewer full-time equivalent workers from 2017 to 2024 (Congressional Budget Office, 2014). Specifically, the CBO wrote:

The reduction in CBO's projections of hours worked represents a decline in the number of full-time-equivalent workers of about 2.0 million in 2017, rising to about 2.5 million in 2024. Although

CBO projects that total employment (and compensation) will increase over the coming decade, that increase will be smaller than it would have been in the absence of the ACA. The decline in fulltime-equivalent employment stemming from the ACA will consist of some people not being employed at all and other people working fewer hours; however, CBO has not tried to quantify those two components of the overall effect. The estimated reduction stems almost entirely from a net decline in the amount of labor that workers choose to supply, rather than from a net drop in businesses' demand for labor, so it will appear almost entirely as a reduction in labor force participation and in hours worked relative to what would have occurred otherwise rather than as an increase in unemployment (that is, more workers seeking but not finding jobs) or underemployment (such as part-time workers who would prefer to work more hours per week). (Congressional Budget Office, 2014)

Opponents of the ACA used this as evidence that the law was reducing employment—including running ads on the topic during the 2014 campaign season (Contorno and Jacobson, 2014). Conservative critics also interpreted the analysis as evidence that the ACA gives individuals an incentive to not work (Rosario, 2014). Meanwhile, the Administration stated that the analysis demonstrated that the ACA gave workers more choices in their employment—and that it gave them greater agency over how much they worked (Furman, 2014; Office of the Press Secretary, 2014). It is clear that the ACA will impact the labor market; however, CBO's analysis indicates that the ACA will not necessarily lead to fewer jobs or greater unemployment, but fewer hours worked due to employee choice.

Overall, it is too early to say that the ACA is leading to increased entrepreneurship and is reducing job lock. However, some of the insurance market reforms in the ACA, as well as the premium subsidies to purchase coverage through the exchanges, may encourage individuals to change jobs or start their own businesses. In particular, requirements that health insurers must cover any applicant and that prohibit denial for preexisting conditions give potential entrepreneurs certainty that they will be able to access coverage without employer-sponsored health plans (Litan, 2014). Over the coming years, the ACA will have many intended and unintended consequences on the labor market. Assessing whether or not it will promote entrepreneurship and reduce a job lock will be difficult to track, but economic theory and early preliminary projections and evidence suggest the law could have a positive impact on the phenomena.

FURTHER READING

Blumberg, L., Corlette, S., and Lucia, K. 2013. "The Affordable Care Act: Improving Incentives for Entrepreneurship and Self-employment." The Center on Health Insurance Reforms, Robert Wood Johnson Foundation, and the Urban Institute. Accessed January 31, 2015. http://www.rwjf.org/content/dam/farm/reports/issue_briefs/2013/rwjf406367.

Chopra, A. 2009. "America's Innovators Call for Health Care Reform to Unlock Jobs of the Future." *The White House Blog.* Accessed January 29, 2015. http://www.whitehouse.gov/blog/2009/12/18/industries-future-weigh-need-health-reform.

Congressional Budget Office. 2014. "Labor Market Effects of the Affordable Care Act: Updated Estimates." Accessed October 6, 2015. http://www.cbo.gov/sites/default/files/cbofiles/attachments/45010-breakout-AppendixC.pdf.

Contorno, S., and Jacobson, L. 2014. "NRCC Says Congressional Budget Office Predicts Obamacare Will Cost Economy 2.5 Million Jobs." Politifact.com. Accessed January 31, 2015. http://www.politifact.com/truth-o-meter/statements/2014/feb/14/national-republican-congressional-committee/nrcc-says-congressional-budget-office-predicts-oba/.

Fairlie, R., Kapur, K., and Gates, S. 2010. "Is Employer-Based Health Insurance a Barrier to Entrepreneurship?" Kaufman-RAND Institute for Entrepreneurship Public Policy. Accessed January 31, 2015. http://www.rand.org/content/dam/rand/pubs/working_papers/2010/RAND_WR637-1.pdf.

Furman, J. 2014. "Six Economic Benefits of the Affordable Care Act." Council of Economic Advisors, The White House. Accessed January 29, 2015. http://www.whitehouse.gov/blog/2014/02/06/six-economic-benefits-affordable-care-act.

Gitis, B. 2014. "The Problem with ACA's 30 Hour Work Week." American Action Forum. Accessed January 3, 2014. http://americanactionforum.org/insights/the-problem-with-acas-30-hour-work-week.

Gonshorowski, D. 2013. "The Affordable Care Act Negatively Impacts the Labor Supply." Heritage Foundation. Accessed January 3, 2015. http://www.heritage.org/research/reports/2013/03/impact-of-the-patient-protecti.

Government Accountability Office. 2011. "Health Care Coverage: Job Lock and the Potential Impact of the Patient Protection and Affordable Care Act." Accessed January 31, 2015. http://www.gao.gov/assets/590/586973.pdf.

H.R. 2520. 2009. "The Patients' Choice Act." Accessed January 31, 2015. http://paulryan.house.gov/uploadedfiles/pcasummary15p.pdf.

Henry J. Henry J. Kaiser Family Foundation and Health Research Educational Trust. 2014. "Employer Health Benefits: 2014 Annual Survey." Accessed January 3, 2015. http://files.kff.org/attachment/2014-employer-health-benefits-survey-full-report.

Litan, R. 2014. "Protecting Entrepreneurs amid a Push for Health-Care Reforms." Brookings. Accessed January 31, 2015. http://www.brookings.edu/research/opinions/2014/12/11-protecting-entrepreneurs-health-care-reforms-litan.

Moffit, R., and Owcharenko, N. 2008. "The McCain Health Care Plan: More Power to Families." The Heritage Foundation. Accessed January 31, 2015. http://www.heritage.org/research/reports/2008/10/the-mccain-health-care-plan-more-power-to-families.

Office of the Press Secretary. 2014. "Statement by the Press Secretary on Today's CBO Report and the Affordable Care Act." The White House. Accessed January 31, 2015. http://www.whitehouse.gov/the-press-office/2014/02/04/statement-press-secretary-today-s-cbo-report-and-affordable-care-act.

Romer, C. 2009. "The Bottom Line on Health Reform and Jobs." *The White House Blog.* Accessed January 29, 2015. http://www.whitehouse.gov/blog/2009/12/09/bottom-line-health-reform-and-jobs.

Rosario, K. 2014. "Obama Administration: Obamacare Means People Can 'Pursue Their Dreams,' Not Work." Heritage Action for America. Accessed January 31, 2015. http://heritageaction.com/2014/02/obama-administration-obamacare-means-people-can-pursue-their-dreams-not-work/.

Tuzeman, D., and Becker, T. 2014. "Does Health-Care Reform Support Self-Employment?" Federal Reserve Bank of Kansas City Economic Review, Third Quarter 2014, 27–45. Accessed May 13, 2015. https://kansascityfed.org/publicat/econrev/pdf/14q3Tuzemen-Becker.pdf.

5

❖❖❖

Coverage for Individuals under the Affordable Care Act

The impacts of a law as complex as the ACA on individuals are difficult to predict and assess, but central to any public debate or discussion of the law. Perhaps the most contentious issue related to impact on individuals has been what the law would mean for health insurance premiums and costs. Supporters of the ACA have made claims about how the law will reduce premiums for health insurance, with the Obama Administration and some health economists citing anywhere from $2,000 to $3,000 in savings for businesses or families. Meanwhile opponents have focused their claims—and evidence—on premiums and costs increasing as a result of the law's coverage and benefit requirements. In particular, Republicans have highlighted the potential for "sticker shock" for younger healthier individuals whose premiums are likely to be higher as a result of the changes in health reform. Both Democrats and Republicans have had difficulty proving their claims on the law's impact on premiums. Unfortunately, many reports fail to provide a complete picture of the cost to individuals, which should take not only premiums into account but also the premium subsidies and cost-sharing reductions most health insurance exchange enrollees are eligible for.

In addition to the issue of the impact of the ACA on premium costs, there is continuing debate on who is eligible for coverage under the law. The claim that the ACA extends coverage to undocumented immigrants has quietly persisted. While the law goes to clear lengths to prohibit and prevent undocumented immigrants from enrolling in coverage, the recent immigration debate and other issues have resulted in this claim resurfacing. This chapter assesses the law's impacts on health insurance premiums, costs to individuals, and who is eligible for coverage through the ACA.

Q25. WILL THE AFFORDABLE CARE ACT REDUCE INSURANCE PREMIUMS, AS MANY ADVOCATES PREDICTED?

Answer: This is a difficult question to answer, because it is impossible to know how much insurance premiums would be if the ACA had not been signed into law. However, some of the more optimistic scenarios projected by ACA advocates, in which they assessed that the ACA could reduce health insurance premiums for many families by $2,000 to $3,000, have not been realized. Meanwhile, partisan arguments over Obamacare's overall impact on premiums has remained heated.

The Facts: A record 50 million Americans were uninsured in 2010 (DeNavas, Proctor, and Smith, 2011). While a number of reasons contributed to the situation, a primary driver of high rates of uninsurance in the United States was the ever-rising costs of health care. One of the critical challenges health reform faces was to expand coverage to the uninsured, but in a sustainable way. As a result, in addition to the coverage expansion, the law included a number of provisions aimed at bending the cost curve in health care. The Administration, Democratic members of Congress, and other supporters of health reform believed that these provisions in the law would reduce the cost of health insurance compared to the status quo (i.e., no health reform). On several occasions, President Obama stated that the law would reduce health care costs for businesses and families, and that large employers could save anywhere from $2,000 to $3,000 per family over time (Obama, 2009, 2011). Health economist David Cutler projected that the law would lower premiums by nearly $2,000 per family relative to the status quo—a number that generated much speculation and controversy (Cutler, Davis, and Stremikis, 2010). However, it has proven difficult to quantify the impact of the myriad provisions in the law, as well as broader economic trends, on the cost of health insurance.

Critics have contended the exact opposite—that health reform will lead to sticker shock—or higher premium prices due to new insurance market reforms and coverage requirements. An analysis by the American Action Forum, a right-leaning think tank, projected that at a minimum, premiums would not drop—and that they could rise by as much as 13 percent (Holtz-Eakin and Parente, 2013). Republican Congressional leaders also claimed that the law would increase premiums—citing Congressional Budget Office (CBO) analyses as evidence (Boehner and McConnell, 2010).

Quantifying the impact of health reform on premiums is difficult, however, with some economists asserting that it is like comparing apples and oranges. Insurance market reforms contained in the ACA ensured that small-group and individual plans sold starting in 2014 would be more comprehensive than some of the "bare bones" policies available prior to passage of Obamacare. As a result, it is difficult to truly project what policies would have cost with or without health reform.

Rising health care costs were a key driver for health reform. By 2009, health care spending had reached $8,175 per capita and accounted for 17.4 percent of United States GDP (Centers for Medicare and Medicaid Services, 2014). Against this backdrop, supporters of health reform sought to address the dual challenges facing the United States health care system—to reduce the uninsured and to bend the cost curve. The two problems went hand in hand, and addressing both was necessary for a more inclusive and sustainable system in the long run.

Gaining political support for health reform required helping those with insurance—and worried about its rising costs—understand the longer-term benefits of reform for them. One potential benefit was lowering the cost growth in health care, which would slow premium growth or increases relative to no health reform. Slower cost growth could occur via two mechanisms: (1) reduced uncompensated care costs as a result of more people having insurance and (2) payment and delivery reforms in the law—both of which the ACA would do. The President and other supporters of the law, including economists, made a number of statements that the ACA was going to reduce health insurance premiums. Some even predicted average premium reductions of $2,000 to 3,000 for many families. In 2011, President Obama gave a speech stating that:

> health insurance reform could save large employers anywhere from $2,000 to $3,000 per family, per year, that they cover in health care costs by 2019. And that's money that businesses can use to grow and invest and to hire. That's money that workers won't have to see vanish from their paychecks or bonuses in the form of higher deductibles or bigger co-payments. That's good for all of us. (The White House, 2011)

A prominent health economist, and supporter of the ACA, released a study projecting that health reform would reduce health care expenditures by nearly $600 billion and lower premiums by $2,000 on average relative to if health reform had not passed—mostly due to payment and delivery reforms and Medicare payment reductions (Cutler, Davis, and Stremikis, 2010). The study tried to project the impact of the law on total health system expenditures, but the projections will take more time to evaluate.

On the other hand, there were numerous studies suggesting the ACA was going to lead to "sticker shock," or significant increases in premiums, especially for younger people on the individual market. Beginning at the very outset of the health reform debate, one management consulting firm released several reports on how the ACA would impact insurance premiums. In 2009, Oliver Wyman released a report projecting that premiums for the youngest 30 percent of people on the individual market would increase by 35 percent on average (Grau and Giesa, 2009). Several reasons for significant premium increases were noted in the report, including the new coverage requirements in the law, and the rating requirements which only allowed insurers to vary rates from 3:1 based on age.

Reports and estimates such as this one quickly became politicized by ACA opponents to assert that President Obama's claim that health reform

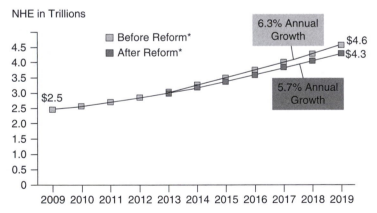

* Estimate of pre-reform national health spending when corrected to reflect underutilization of services by previously uninsured.
Data: Authors' estimates.

Figure 5.1 Total National Health Expenditures (NHE), 2009–2019 before and after Reform

Source: Cutler, D., Davis, K., and Stremikis, K. 2010. "The Impact of Health Reform on Health System Spending." The Commonwealth Fund. Accessed February 5, 2015. http://www.commonwealthfund.org/~/media/Files/Publications/Issue%20Brief/2010/May/1405_Cutler_impact_hlt_reform_on_hlt_sys_spending_ib_v4.pdf.

would reduce premiums was wrong. In 2013, Republican members of key House and Senate Congressional committees released a report summarizing studies and statements that supported their point of the view that the ACA would increase premiums. The report warned:

> At a time of negative economic growth and sluggish job creation, middle class families are struggling to make ends meet. Higher health care premiums are the last thing single young adults and working families can afford. Yet contrary to what the president promised, that is exactly what Obamacare is projected to do. (House Committee on Energy and Commerce et al., 2013)

The phenomenon of sticker shock would be expected to be strongest in 2014, when the new market reforms and rating rules went into effect. The American Action Forum projected that no one would see premiums decrease starting 2014—and that for some Americans, premiums would remain the same or increase (Holtz-Eakin and Parente, 2013). However, none of these analyses took into account the impact of health insurance subsidies on individual premium payments.

In 2009 during the health reform debate, CBO analyzed the likely impacts of the ACA on health insurance premiums. CBO took into account the effects of the insurance market reforms, of pooling risk in the individual market, and of health insurance subsidies for individuals and families from 100 to 400 percent of the Federal Poverty Level. CBO projected the following:

> CBO and JCT estimate that the average premium per person covered (including dependents) for new nongroup policies would be about 10 percent to 13 percent higher in 2016 than the average premium for nongroup coverage in that same year under current law. About half of those enrollees would receive government subsidies that would reduce their costs well below the premiums that would be charged for such policies under current law. (Congressional Budget Office, 2009)

CBO projected that in total, after taking into account the higher levels of coverage required by the ACA, the impacts of pooling risk, new individuals entering the market, and health insurance premium subsidies, individuals would pay 56 to 59 percent less than if the ACA did not become law (Congressional Budget Office, 2009). Given that most people purchasing individual insurance policies through the new health insurance exchanges would receive subsidies, not taking them into account in any discussion of sticker shock fails to account for the actual cost or impact to individuals, which would be to reduce the relative cost of insurance.

The evidence does not suggest that on its own the ACA has lowered premiums or premium cost growth; however, it is noteworthy that widespread increases in year over year insurance costs have not been observed from 2014 to 2015. A Henry J. Kaiser Family Foundation report found a slight premium decrease of 0.8 percent for "silver" coverage plans in 16 cities (Cox et al., 2015). CBO's estimates of the overall costs of the coverage expansion have also been relatively stable, although in 2015 CBO projected a 20 percent decrease relative to its 2014 estimate in the 10-year cost of the premium subsidies and other cost-sharing reductions (Congressional Budget Office, 2015a). The drop is partially attributed to slower-than-expected growth in premium costs (Congressional Budget Office, 2015b). While quantifying the exact impact of the ACA in total on premiums is difficult and will take longer to assess, the early evidence suggests slower than historical growth and stable premiums in the exchanges.

FURTHER READING

Boehner, J., and McConnell, M. 2010. "The President Could Have Chosen a Bipartisan Approach." *Wall Street Journal*, March 15, 2010. Accessed February 5, 2015. http://www.speaker.gov/op-ed/obamacare-and-buzzsaw-opposition-boehner-and-mcconnell-op-ed-wsj#sthash.JqNxvXgY.dpuf.

Centers for Medicare and Medicaid Services. 2014. "The National Health Expenditure Accounts, Table 1. National Health Expenditures; Aggregate and Per Capita Amounts, Annual Percent Change and Percent Distribution: Selected Calendar Years 1960–2013." Accessed February 5, 2015. http://www.cms.gov/Research-Statistics-Data-and-Systems/Statistics-Trends-and-Reports/NationalHealthExpendData/NationalHealthAccountsHistorical.html.

Congressional Budget Office. 2009. "An Analysis of Health Insurance Premiums under the Patient Protection and Affordable Care Act." Accessed February 25, 2015. http://www.cbo.gov/sites/default/files/11-30-premiums.pdf.

Congressional Budget Office. 2015a. "Insurance Coverage Provisions of the Affordable Care Act—CBO's March 2015 Baseline." Accessed March 10, 2015. http://www.cbo.gov/sites/default/files/cbofiles/attachments/43900-2015-03-ACAtables.pdf.

Congressional Budget Office. 2015b. "Updated Budget Projections: 2015 to 2025." Accessed March 10, 2015. http://www.cbo.gov/sites/default/files/cbofiles/attachments/49973-Updated_Budget_Projections.pdf.

Cox, C., Levitt, L., Claxton, G., Ma, R., and Duddy-Tenbrunsel, R. 2015. "Analysis of 2015 Premium Changes in the Affordable Care Act's Health Insurance Marketplaces." Henry J. Kaiser Family Foundation. Accessed February 25, 2015. http://files.kff.org/attachment/analysis-of-2015-premium-changes-in-the-affordable-care-acts-health-insurance-marketplaces-issue-brief.

Cutler, D., Davis, K., and Stremikis, K. 2010. "The Impact of Health Reform on Health System Spending." The Commonwealth Fund. Accessed February 5, 2015. http://www.commonwealthfund.org/~/media/Files/Publications/Issue%20Brief/2010/May/1405_Cutler_impact_hlt_re form_on_hlt_sys_spending_ib_v4.pdf.

DeNavas, C., Proctor, B., and Smith, J. 2011. "Income, Poverty, and Health Insurance Coverage in the United States: 2010." United States Census Bureau. Accessed February 28, 2015. http://www.census.gov/prod/2011pubs/p60-239.pdf.

Grau, J., and Giesa, K. 2009. "Impact of the Patient Protection and Affordable Care Act on Costs in the Individual and Small-Employer Health Insurance Markets." Oliver Wyman. Accessed February 25, 2015. http://www.oliverwyman.com/content/dam/oliver-wyman/global/en/files/archive/2009/YBS009-11-28_PPACA120309.pdf.

Holtz-Eakin, D., and Parente, S. 2013. "Individual and Small Group Insurance Premiums and the Affordable Care Act: Analytic Results." American Action Forum. Accessed February 5, 2015. http://americanactionforum.org/sites/default/files/Premiums%20and%20ACA%20Analytics.pdf.

House Committee on Energy and Commerce, Majority Staff, Senate Committee on Finance, Minority Staff, and Senate Committee on Health, Education, Labor and Pensions, Minority Staff. 2013. "The Price of Obamacare's Broken Promises: Young Adults and Middle Class Families Set to Endure Higher Premiums and Unaffordable Coverage." Accessed February 25, 2015. http://energycommerce.house.gov/sites/republicans.energycommerce.house.gov/files/analysis/20130305PremiumReport.pdf.

The White House. 2009. "Remarks by the President after Meeting with Senate Democrats." The White House, Office of the Press Secretary. Accessed February 5, 2015. http://www.whitehouse.gov/the-press-office/remarks-president-after-meeting-with-senate-democrats.

The White House. 2011. "Remarks by the President at Families USA Health Action Conference." The White House, Office of the Press Secretary. Accessed February 5, 2015. http://www.whitehouse.gov/the-press-office/2011/01/28/remarks-president-families-usa-health-action-conference.

Q26. WILL THE AFFORDABLE CARE ACT INCREASE HEALTH CARE COSTS FOR YOUNGER, HEALTHIER INDIVIDUALS?

Answer: One of the most frequent criticisms of the ACA is that it increases health care costs for younger, healthier individuals due to new premium rating rules. Critics of the law contended that the new require-ments in the law to offer coverage to all individuals regardless of pre-existing conditions, and limitations on how much insurers could vary premiums based on age, would drive up prices. In particular, ACA oppo-nents and insurers charged that young people—who needed to enroll in the exchange-based plans—would experience "sticker shock" in 2014 (America's Health Insurance Plans, 2013; House Committee on Energy and Commerce et al., 2013). However, the ACA's impact on young adults has been far more complex. While the rating rules increased costs of coverage—without taking into account the counteracting effects of the premium subsidies—there were new provisions in the law that expanded coverage. These provisions were especially critical to young adults, who historically have had the highest insurance rates of insurance—and the lowest rates of coverage—of American age groups. In total, the ACA has had positive impacts on young adults, more of whom have health insur-ance with a basic set of benefits.

The Facts: The ACA included a combination of insurance market reforms and new rules limiting how insurers can vary their premiums for individuals. For instance, the law required that insurance companies had to cover anyone seeking to enroll in a plan—a mandate known as "guar-anteed issue." The ACA also prohibited insurers from denying coverage to anyone with a preexisting condition. In addition to these insurance market reforms, which were aimed at guaranteeing that policies be made available to anyone wishing to purchase coverage, the ACA limited how much insurers could vary premiums based on certain factors. For example, the ACA prohibited varying premiums based on health status or gender. Premium variations based on age were allowed but were limited to 3:1—so that the premiums for older individuals cannot be more than three times that for younger individuals. Before the new ACA rating rules went into effect in 2014, typical variations were 5:1 (Levitt, Claxton, and Dam-ico, 2013). The more limited premium variation bands generally increase costs for younger individuals and decrease costs for older individuals.

In this system, younger individuals are subsidizing the medical costs of older individuals—with the idea that eventually as they age they would benefit from the same cross-subsidization. However, to maintain affordable premiums in the reformed individual market where all lives are in a single risk pool, sufficient numbers of young people must enroll in coverage. Otherwise, premiums would become increasingly expensive, likely driving more young people out of the market and making premiums unsustainable for those remaining. This phenomenon is sometimes called an insurance death spiral.

A Henry J. Kaiser Family Foundation analysis projected that 40 percent of those enrolled in new exchange plans would need to be young adults, underscoring how critical the group is to the success of the ACA's exchanges and insurance market reforms (Levitt, Claxton, and Damico, 2013). However, from the start of the health reform debate, insurers, as well as critics of the effort, expressed concern about how the limitations on age-based premium variation would increase costs for young adults and discourage their enrollment in the reformed market.

For instance, GOP members of the main Congressional Committees that oversee health care issues and programs wrote in a jointly released report:

> RATE SHOCK FOR YOUNG AMERICANS. Obamacare failed to address the relationship between premium increases and health insurance costs in the United States. Premiums continue to be based on the growth in health care spending and government rules that govern insurance rates. Since Obamacare imposed several new regulations that make coverage unaffordable, premiums will only grow further out of control. In the case of young adults, the premium spike will be even more painful. (House Committee on Energy and Commerce et al., 2013)

The warnings of sticker shock were rooted in a number of actuarial and management consulting reports citing the increased costs of health insurance—especially for young adults—once the ACA's market reforms went into effect. One analysis noted that premiums for individuals aged 21 to 29 years would increase by 42 percent compared to if the ACA had never gone into effect (Giesa and Carlson, 2013). However, these are national averages—actual increases (or decreases in some states) varied widely depending on what the rating rules in a given state were before 2014. Insurers expressed serious concern that these types of rate increases relative to the pre-ACA individual insurance market would result in young people dropping coverage or not even enrolling in the new exchange-based plans—thereby increasing costs for others (America's Health Insurance Plans, 2013).

However, these reports sounding the alarm about giant premium increases for young people do not take into account the impact of the premium subsidies, which were not previously available to anyone on the individual (or any other) market. One report found that subsidies could decrease the cost of coverage anywhere from 40 to 94 percent depending on income (O'Connor, 2013). To assess individuals' true out-of-pocket costs for health insurance, which is often the deciding factor in whether or not to enroll in coverage, these subsidies must be taken into account.

On the other hand, the ACA also included provisions that increased coverage for young adults. In 2009, 31.4 percent of individuals 19 to 25 years of age were uninsured—the highest percentage of any age group (DeNavas, Proctor, and Smith, 2011). Young adults are at particular risk for being uninsured for many reasons. One major factor is that coverage through public programs, such as Medicaid, or through their parents' employer-sponsored insurance, ended at 19 or 21 years of age. Young people are also more likely to have part-time jobs or work in industry sectors that do not offer health insurance at all.

With this in mind, the architects of the ACA included a provision that required insurers to allow young adults up to 26 years of age to remain on their parents' health insurance plans starting in November 2010. By the end of 2011, estimates suggested that over 3 million young adults had gained coverage through this provision of Obamacare (Sommers, 2012). By 2013, the percentage of those uninsured in this age group had fallen to 22.6—a staggering drop, especially given that it occurred even before the health insurance exchanges and premium subsidies had taken effect (Smith and Medalia, 2014). This provision was quite successful in extending coverage to young adults—many of whom may have remained uninsured otherwise.

Democrats seized on this data to demonstrate a tangible benefit of the law in advance of the exchanges and insurance subsidies in 2014. For instance, Chairman Tom Harkin (D-IA) of the Health, Education, Labor and Pensions (HELP) Committee stated at a hearing:

> Before the Affordable Care Act, millions of young adults went without health insurance because their jobs didn't offer it, or because they were ineligible for coverage on their parents' policy. These young people—starting a new job or a new business, folks who don't have a lot of money—had to largely fend for themselves in a chaotic, unregulated market for individual coverage that charges high premiums for only modest benefits. Now, health reform allows these young people—more than 2 million of them—to stay on their parents'

policy until age 26. This reform relieves young people of the burden of high health insurance costs—and for those who can't afford coverage, the fear of financial ruin. This reform is particularly important for young people with chronic illness. (Harkin, 2011)

On January 1, 2014, the ACA's health insurance exchanges and premium subsidies went into effect. One of the most concerning issues was whether young adults would enroll in the new coverage options. Their robust participation was critical so that sicker individuals with unmet health needs could purchase coverage. Otherwise, the aforementioned insurance death spiral might take hold and threaten the financial underpinnings of the reforms.

As of April 2014, the end of the first open enrollment period for exchanges, young adults aged 18 to 34 years accounted for 28 percent of the 8 million enrolled (Assistant Secretary for Planning and Evaluation, 2014). Over 2 million young adults gained coverage in the first year of open enrollment, with many receiving subsidies to pay for their exchange-based coverage. One report from the left-leaning Center for American Progress estimated that only 3 percent of young adults would

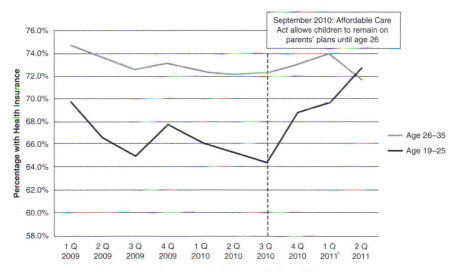

Figure 5.2 Percentage of Young Adults with Health Insurance, 2009–2011 by Quarter and Age Group

Source: Sommers, B. 2012. "Number of Young Adults Gaining Insurance Due to the Affordable Care Act Now Tops 3 Million." Assistant Secretary for Planning and Evaluation, Department of Health and Human Services. Accessed February 28, 2015. http://aspe.hhs.gov/aspe/gaininginsurance/rb.cfm.

experience higher premiums in the individual market because they would not receive premium subsidies to offset any relative increase in premium costs due to the ACA (Calsyn and Rosenthal, 2013). While it is difficult to assess what the impact of premium changes was on young adults' willingness to enroll in coverage, it is clear that multiple provisions in the ACA increased coverage for this vulnerable age group.

Finally, while the percentage of exchange enrollees who were young adults fell short of the Henry J. Kaiser Family Foundation's projected need of 40 percent, premiums did not rise significantly on average across the country in 2015 (Levitt, Claxton, and Damico, 2013). In fact, another Henry J. Kaiser Family Foundation report found a slight decrease of 0.8 percent for silver plans on overage in 16 cities (Cox et al., 2015). The concerns over sticker shock had merit—even if some of the charges were politically motivated—as premiums for young adults on average are higher starting 2014 than before the ACA's market reforms and rating rules went into effect. However, taking into account the premium subsidies and the provision to allow individuals up to 26 years to remain on their parents' insurance plans, the ACA's overall effect on young adults has been positive.

FURTHER READING

America's Health Insurance Plans. 2013. "New Study Finds ACA's Age Rating Restrictions Will Increase Premiums for Younger Individuals." Accessed February 28, 2015. http://www.ahip.org/News/Press-Room/2013/New-Study-Finds-ACA-s-Age-Rating-Restrictions-will-Increase-Premiums-for-Younger-Individuals.aspx.

Assistant Secretary for Planning and Evaluation. 2014. "Health Insurance Marketplace: Summary Enrollment Report for the Initial Annual Open Enrollment Period." Department of Health and Human Services. Accessed February 28, 2015. http://aspe.hhs.gov/health/reports/2014/MarketPlaceEnrollment/Apr2014/ib_2014Apr_enrollment.pdf.

Calsyn, M., and Rosenthal, L. 2013. "How the Affordable Care Act Helps Young Adults." Center for American Progress. Accessed February 28, 2015. https://www.americanprogress.org/issues/health care/report/2013/05/20/63792/how-the-affordable-care-act-helps-young-adults/.

Cox, C., Levitt, L., Claxton, G., et al. 2015. "Analysis of 2015 Premium Changes in the Affordable Care Act's Health Insurance Marketplaces."

Henry J. Kaiser Family Foundation. Accessed February 25, 2015. http://files.kff.org/attachment/analysis-of-2015-premium-changes-in-the-affordable-care-acts-health-insurance-marketplaces-issue-brief.

DeNavas, C., Proctor, B., and Smith, J. 2011. "Income, Poverty, and Health Insurance Coverage in the United States: 2010." United States Census Bureau. Accessed February 28, 2015. http://www.census.gov/prod/2011pubs/p60-239.pdf.

Giesa, K., and Carlson, C. 2013. "Age Band Compression under Health Care Reform." Accessed October 8, 2015. http://www.nahu.org/meetings/capitol/2013/attendees/jumpdrive/contingencies20130102_1357146485000c7cc7dd5e1_pp.pdf.

Harkin, T. 2011. "Hearing on the Affordable Care Act: The Impact of Health Insurance Reform on Health Care Consumers." Accessed October 8, 2015. http://www.help.senate.gov/ranking/newsroom/press/help-committee-hears-from-americans-on-health-reform-benefits.

House Committee on Energy and Commerce, Majority Staff, Senate Committee on Finance, Minority Staff, and Senate Committee on Health, Education, Labor and Pensions, Minority Staff. 2013. "The Price of Obamacare's Broken Promises: Young Adults and Middle Class Families Set to Endure Higher Premiums and Unaffordable Coverage." Accessed February 25, 2015. http://energycommerce.house.gov/sites/republicans.energycommerce.house.gov/files/analysis/20130305PremiumReport.pdf.

Levitt, L., Claxton, G., and Damico, A. 2013. "The Numbers behind the 'Young Invincibles' and the Affordable Care Act." Henry J. Kaiser Family Foundation. Accessed February 28, 2015. http://kff.org/health-reform/perspective/the-numbers-behind-young-invincibles-and-the-affordable-care-act/.

O'Connor, J. 2013. "Comprehensive Assessment of ACA Factors That Will Affect Individual Market Premiums in 2014." Milliman. Accessed February 28, 2015. http://ahip.org/MillimanReportACA2013/.

Smith, J., and Medalia, C. 2014. "Health Insurance Coverage in the United States: 2013." United States Census Bureau. Accessed February 28, 2015. http://www.census.gov/content/dam/Census/library/publications/2014/demo/p60-250.pdf.

Sommers, B. 2012. "Number of Young Adults Gaining Insurance Due to the Affordable Care Act Now Tops 3 Million." Assistant Secretary for Planning and Evaluation, Department of Health and Human Services. Accessed February 28, 2015. http://aspe.hhs.gov/aspe/gaininginsurance/rb.cfm.

Q27. DOES THE AFFORDABLE CARE ACT PROVIDE HEALTH COVERAGE TO UNDOCUMENTED IMMIGRANTS?

Answer: No. The Affordable Care Act states in multiple places that only United States citizens and legal residents are eligible to enroll in the ACA's health insurance exchanges and receive subsidies to help pay for their policies.

The Facts: As the debate over health reform began in earnest in 2009, one of the early myths that surfaced was how the law would treat undocumented immigrants. Even before passage of health reform legislation in the House or the Senate, reports circulated, especially in conservative media circles, that undocumented immigrants would be able to access health insurance subsidies and other benefits if Obamacare was passed into law. While the origins of the myth are not clear, it has persisted over the past several years. In the summer of 2009, PolitiFact.com debunked the myth that undocumented immigrants would receive health care services for free via an e-mail that was circulating whose origins were unknown, but tied to a conservative writer (Holan, 2009).

Since then, the myth has persisted for several reasons. First, over five months after open enrollment ended for the 2014 plan year, the Department of Health and Human Services asked nearly 1 million enrollees for immigration documentation; however, 115,000 did not respond to the request (Centers for Medicare and Medicaid Services, 2014). Conservatives alleged that this proved undocumented immigrants had received ACA benefits. Second, as President Obama's executive orders related to immigration went into effect, prominent Republicans made unfounded charges that the administration was giving health care coverage to undocumented immigrants (Miller, 2014). Republican Senator David Vitter (R-LA), for example, asserted that

> the Obama administration is bending over backwards to give Obamacare to illegal immigrants but won't protect hardworking American citizens who are losing their health care coverage. . . . The Obama administration has been granting deadline extensions, making excuses and turning a blind eye to falsified documents by illegal immigrants. . . . Enough is enough, and they need to provide answers to why they think illegal immigrants should be eligible for Obamacare. (Miller, 2014)

However, the ACA clearly states that undocumented individuals cannot enroll in coverage through the health insurance exchanges and that any immigration-related executive orders do not change or affect ACA eligibility.

The ACA expanded coverage to the uninsured via the Medicaid expansion and the establishment of new exchanges where qualifying individuals and families could use premium subsidies to purchase insurance coverage. The controversy around undocumented immigrants obtaining coverage centered on the new source of coverage—the exchanges. However, the ACA states in multiples places that only U.S. citizens and legal residents were eligible to enroll in exchange coverage and receive a subsidy in multiple sections, as illustrated here:

    (b) Information Required To Be Provided by Applicants—
        (1) IN GENERAL—An applicant for enrollment in a qualified health plan offered through an Exchange in the individual market shall provide. . .
        (2) CITIZENSHIP OR IMMIGRATION STATUS—The following information shall be provided with respect to every enrollee:
            (A) In the case of an enrollee whose eligibility is based on an attestation of citizenship of the enrollee, the enrollee's social security number.
            (B) In the case of an individual whose eligibility is based on an attestation of the enrollee's immigration status, the enrollee's social security number (if applicable) and such identifying information with respect to the enrollee's immigration status as the Secretary, after consultation with the Secretary of Homeland Security, determines appropriate. (H.R. 3590, 2010)

Even though passage of the law and its clear language should have put the myth to rest, it has continued to resurface.

In 2014, the health insurance exchanges launched with nearly 8 million individuals enrolling in coverage during the first open enrollment period. However, five months after open enrollment ended, HHS sent notices out to 966,000 individuals asking them to submit documentation on their immigration status (Centers for Medicare and Medicaid Services, 2014). Nearly 90 percent of individuals responded, but termination notices were sent to the 115,000 people who did not respond to requests for immigration status information (Centers for Medicare and Medicaid Services, 2014). However, the Department's notice reignited charges that the ACA provided benefits and coverage to undocumented immigrants.

Oregon also made headlines when the state's malfunctioning exchange enrolled 4,000 undocumented immigrants in a state program providing pregnancy services into ACA coverage (Budnick, 2014). In the end, the Department terminated coverage for those that did not supply the appropriate paperwork and Oregon corrected the incorrect enrollment, but the allegations that benefits were being extended to undocumented immigrants would continue to resurface.

In November 2014, nearly a year after the ACA coverage expansion launched, President Obama issued an executive order on several immigration issues. One of the most controversial provisions in the executive order allowed undocumented immigrants that met a number of criteria, including having been in the country for more than five years, having children who are U.S. citizens or legal residents, and passage of a criminal background check, to apply to stay in the United States without being deported (White House, 2014). In a speech announcing the new policy, President Obama made clear that it did not confer benefits that U.S. citizens receive on these individuals:

> Now, let's be clear about what it [the executive order] isn't. This deal does not apply to anyone who has come to this country recently. It does not apply to anyone who might come to America illegally in the future. It does not grant citizenship, or the right to stay here permanently, or offer the same benefits that citizens receive—only Congress can do that. All we're saying is we're not going to deport you. (The White House, 2014)

Despite the clarity of the language in the order itself and the President's statements, ACA critics seized on the immigration executive order to allege that ACA benefits would be available to the undocumented immigrants (Uwimana, 2014). At the same time, other ACA opponents were making the exact opposite argument. They alleged that because the undocumented immigrants affected by the executive order would be ineligible for ACA coverage, employers would actually have an incentive to hire them over legal residents and citizens because of the employer responsibility provisions in the law (Dinan, 2014). Employers with 50 or more full-time workers are required to provide affordable coverage, or are subject to a $3,000 penalty per worker that obtains subsidies and coverage through the exchanges. ACA opponents seized on the executive order to make contradictory claims about its relation to health reform.

One of the impacts of deportation fears has been to dampen enrollment of legal Hispanic residents in the ACA's coverage expansion for fear that undocumented family members could be discovered. Unfortunately, Hispanic Americans are at greater risk for developing long-term and chronic health issues, with many not having access to insurance. In 2013, 24 percent of Hispanics in the United States were uninsured—the highest of any racial group (Smith and Medalia, 2014). Hispanic Americans also have higher rates and risks of a number of health problems. For instance, approximately 32 percent of Hispanics have obesity, compared to 26 percent of white Americans (Centers for Disease Control and Prevention, 2012).

Given the high rate of uninsured Hispanic Americans and their health profiles, there have been significant efforts to target them for enrollment in coverage. In June 2014, HHS announced that the uninsured rates among Hispanic Americans fell by 7.7 percent—a significant decrease; however, approximately 34 percent still remained uninsured (Finegold and Gunja, 2014). Even though the ACA nor subsequent Administration actions do not extend coverage to undocumented immigrants, the two topics have become linked.

FURTHER READING

Budnick, N. 2014. "Cover Oregon Health Insurance Exchange Fiasco Spawns Problems for Low-Income Oregonians' Health Plan." *The Oregonian*, March 1, 2014. Accessed March 8, 2015. http://www.oregon live.com/health/index.ssf/2014/03/cover_oregon_health_insurance_1 .html.

Centers for Disease Control and Prevention. 2011. "Deaths: Final Data for 2009." National Vital Statistics Reports Volume 60, Number 3. Accessed March 8, 2015. http://www.cdc.gov/nchs/data/nvsr/nvsr60/ nvsr60_03.pdf.

Centers for Disease Control and Prevention. 2012. "Summary Health Statistics for U.S. Adults: National Health Interview Survey, 2010." Vital and Health Statistics, Series 10, Number 252. Accessed March 8, 2015. http://www.cdc.gov/nchs/data/series/sr_10/sr10_252.pdf.

Centers for Medicare and Medicaid Services. 2014. "Press Release: CMS Update on Consumers Who Have Data Matching Issues." Accessed March 4, 2015. http://www.cms.gov/Newsroom/MediaReleaseDatabase/ Press-releases/2014-Press-releases-items/2014-09-15.html.

Dinan, S. 2014. "Obamacare Offers Firms $3,000 Incentive to Hire Illegals over Native-Born Workers." The *Washington Times*, November 25, 2014. Accessed March 8, 2015. http://www.washingtontimes .com/news/2014/nov/25/obama-amnesty-obamacare-clash-businesses-have-3000/#ixzz3TGzlx2pT.

Finegold, K. and Gunja, M. 2014. "Survey Data on Health Insurance Coverage for 2013 and 2014." Assistant Secretary for Planning and Evaluation. Department of Health and Human Services. Accessed March 8, 2015. http://aspe.hhs.gov/health/reports/2014/InsuranceEsti mates/ib_InsuranceEstimates.pdf.

Holan, A. 2009. "Email 'Analysis' of Health Bill Needs a Check-up." PolitiFact.com. *Tampa Bay Times*, July, 30, 2009. Accessed March 3, 2015. http://www.politifact.com/truth-o-meter/article/2009/jul/30/ e-mail-analysis-health-bill-needs-check-/.

H.R. 3590. 2010. "Text of the Patient Protection and Affordable Care Act." Accessed March 4, 2015. http://www.gpo.gov/fdsys/pkg/BILLS-111hr3590enr/pdf/BILLS-111hr3590enr.pdf

Miller, S. 2014. "GOP: Obamacare 'Bending over Backwards' for Illegals." *Washington Times*, September 22, 2014. Accessed March 3, 2015. http:// www.washingtontimes.com/news/2014/sep/22/1-million-people-o n-obamacare-fail-to-prove-citize/.

Smith, J., and Medalia, C. 2014. "Health Insurance Coverage in the United States: 2013." United States Census Bureau. Accessed February 28, 2015. http://www.census.gov/content/dam/Census/library/publications/ 2014/demo/p60-250.pdf.

Uwimana, S. 2014. "Laura Ingraham Still Pushing Myth That Undocumented Immigrants Get Obamacare." Media Matters for America. Accessed March 8, 2015. http://mediamatters.org/blog/2014/03/07/ laura-ingraham-still-pushing-myth-that-undocume/198408.

White House. 2014. "Remarks by the President in Address to the National on Immigration." Accessed March 8, 2015. http://www.whitehouse.gov/ issues/immigration/immigration-action#.

Q28. WAS THE "NAVIGATOR" PROGRAM ESTABLISHED IN THE AFFORDABLE CARE ACT TO HELP INDIVIDUALS ENROLL IN THE EXCHANGES EFFECTIVE?

Answer: As with many aspects of the ACA, views differ markedly depending on one's political orientation. Navigators have helped millions of Americans enroll in the insurance exchanges created by the ACA.

However, funding shortfalls, concerns that these "consumer assisters" might compromise personal health information, and operational roadblocks imposed by Republican officials at the state level all reduced the operational effectiveness of this program.

The Facts: The ACA established a Navigator program to help individuals enroll in ACA's exchange-based coverage. The Navigator program was explicitly designed to perform the following functions: (1) to help consumers determine if they are eligible for premium subsidies to purchase exchange coverage, (2) to help them choose and enroll in coverage, (3) to perform outreach and education about the ACA's exchanges, and (4) to refer exchange consumers to the appropriate entity in the event of complaints or questions (Centers for Medicare and Medicaid Services, 2014a).

Official ACA navigators and in-person assisters were all required to complete official trainings before assisting consumers. In order to determine eligibility and support enrollment, however, Navigators and other assisters must collect personal and financial information. This information was necessary to help individuals select the policies that worked best for them, but this aspect of the program raised concerns about ensuring that data are confidential and handled appropriately.

Opponents of the ACA raised concerns about the Navigators and in-person assisters, and many states took steps to regulate their activities. A group of conservative State Attorney Generals wrote to then Secretary of HHS Kathleen Sebelius outlining a number of concerns about the department's regulations for the assister programs. They charged that the program was married by inadequate training, insufficient consumer protections, and additional screening for those certified to assist consumers (State of West Virginia Office of the Attorney General, 2013). Some states also considered and passed legislation requiring background checks for assisters or other requirements to address concerns. Republican members of Congress also weighed in. One of the most prominent efforts was a House Committee on Oversight and Government Reform report on "serious mismanagement of . . . outreach programs exposes Americans to fraud" (House Committee on Oversight and Government Reform, 2013a).

Assisters ended up playing a critical role during the 2014 open enrollment period. There were 28,000 full-time equivalent assisters that helped 10.6 million people (Pollitz, Tolbert, and Ma, 2014). Evidence of fraud and abuse has been limited, and assisters will continue to play an important education and enrollment role in the coming years.

Navigators were to be made available in all states, and funded using federal money, but Congressional opposition to the ACA limited the funds HHS had to distribute across all 50 states. The Administration had to make what ended up being a controversial decision. In 2013, they allocated $54 million from a Congressionally established Prevention and Public Health Trust Fund to operate Navigator programs (Centers for Medicare and Medicaid Services, 2013). For the 2014–2015 open enrollment period, funding totaled $60 million (Centers for Medicare and Medicaid Services, 2014a). However, this level of funding was well below what would be needed to successfully enroll millions of Americans into coverage.

Due to funding and the different state needs depending on the type of exchange model operating, the Administration established two additional consumer assister types—non-Navigator assistance personnel (or in-person assistance personnel) and certified application counselors. The former play a similar role to that of Navigators but are funded through state exchanges (Centers for Medicare and Medicaid Services, 2014b). Certified application counselors perform similar functions as well but are usually provider based and do not receive federal or exchange funds (Centers for Medicare and Medicaid Services, 2014b). The lack of stable Congressional funding and the new consumer assister programs not established in the ACA gave opponents of the law another target for undermining public trust and support in the implementation efforts.

One of the most prominent examples of this line of attack was the 2013 Republican-led House Committee on Oversight and Government Reform report on the Navigator program. The Committee released a report citing numerous violations or inadequate training of consumer assisters—in many cases based on media reports (House Committee on Oversight and Government Reform, 2013a). The reported stated:

> Information obtained from the November 21, 2013 briefing and internal HHS documents call into question the effectiveness of these outreach programs, and, more importantly, the Administration's ability to safeguard consumer information. This update to the Committee's preliminary staff report shows that HHS's mismanagement of the Navigator and Assister programs induces fraudulent behavior and poses real threats to the safety of consumers' personally identifiable information, such as ones social security number, yearly income and other sensitive tax information. (House Committee on Oversight and Government Reform, 2013b)

However, the report relied on HHS documentation, a briefing with senior CMS officials, and media reports to make its conclusions on the effectiveness and integrity of the Navigator program. Attorney Generals from 13 states (primarily so-called Red States led by Republicans) also came together to send Secretary Sebelius a letter detailing a number of concerns about regulations on consumer assister programs. In particular, they called for increased training for consumer assisters, greater levels of consumer protections commensurate with regulations for insurance agents and brokers, and the need for background checks and screening of assisters (State of West Virginia Office of the Attorney General, 2013). Finally, states also enacted new laws or regulations to address some of these gaps, such as requiring background checks and additional licensing and fees (StateReforum, 2014). While some of these measures were intended to protect consumers, some were also politically motivated, with most of the new laws and regulations originating in Republican-led states that were largely opposed to ACA implementation. The speed with which HHS had to stand programs up in 2013 in time for the first 2014 open enrollment, coupled with the political divide over the ACA, made the consumer assister programs another target for controversy.

One of the only evaluations of the exchanges assister programs was conducted in 2014 after open enrollment ended. The Henry J. Kaiser Family Foundation surveyed all consumer assister program directors. In total, there were 4,400 assister programs across the United States that employed the equivalent of 28,000 full-time consumer assisters who are estimated to have helped 10.6 million people during the 2013–2014 open enrollment period (Pollitz, Tolbert, and Ma, 2014). Forty percent of programs reported that they could not help everyone who was seeking assistance, and a small percentage—12 percent—reported that demand for assister services "far outpaced capacity" (Pollitz, Tolbert, and Ma, 2014). Consumer assisters will continue to play a large role in enrolling new individuals into exchange-based coverage, as well as helping people re-enroll in coverage over the next several years. While there were limited media reports of consumer assisters not adhering to regulations and training parameters, widespread problems were not reported.

FURTHER READING

Centers for Medicare and Medicaid Services. 2013. "New Funding Opportunity Announcement for Navigators in Federally-Facilitated and

State Partnership Marketplaces." Accessed March 8, 2015. http://www
.cms.gov/CCIIO/Resources/Fact-Sheets-and-FAQs/navigator-foa.html.

Centers for Medicare and Medicaid Services. 2014a. "Press Release:
CMS Announces Opportunity to Apply for Navigator Grants in
Federally-Facilitated and State Partnership Marketplaces." Accessed
March 8, 2015. http://www.cms.gov/Newsroom/MediaReleaseDatabase/
Press-releases/2014-Press-releases-items/2014-06-10.html.

Centers for Medicare and Medicaid Services. 2014b. "Ways to Help Con-
sumers Apply and Enroll in Health Coverage through the Marketplace."
Accessed March 8, 2015. http://www.cms.gov/CCIIO/Resources/
Fact-Sheets-and-FAQs/Downloads/AssistanceRoles_06-10-14-508.pdf.

House Committee on Oversight and Government Reform. 2013a. "Oversight Report on Obamacare Navigator Program Reveals Mismanagement and Lax Oversight." Accessed March 8, 2015. http://oversight.house
.gov/release/oversight-report-obamacare-navigator-program-reveals-
mismanagement-lax-oversight/.

House Committee on Oversight and Government Reform. 2013b. "Risks
of Fraud and Misinformation with ObamaCare Outreach Campaign:
How Navigator and Assister Program Mismanagement Endangers
Consumers ObamaCare Navigator and Assister Staff Report No. 2."
Accessed March 8, 2015. http://oversight.house.gov/wp-content/
uploads/2013/12/Navigator-Report-Number-Two-12-13-13.pdf.

Pollitz, K., Tolbert, J., and Ma, R. 2014. "Survey of Health Insurance
Marketplace Assister Programs." Henry J. Kaiser Family Foundation.
Accessed March 8, 2015. http://kff.org/health-reform/report/survey-o
f-health-insurance-marketplace-assister-programs/.

State of West Virginia Office of the Attorney General. 2013. "A Com-
munication from the States of West Virginia, Alabama, Florida, Geor-
gia, Kansas, Louisiana, Michigan, Montana, Nebraska, North Dakota,
Oklahoma, South Carolina, and Texas Regarding Data Privacy Risks
Posed by Programs Assisting Consumers with Enrollment in Health
Insurance through the New Exchanges." Accessed March 8, 2015.
http://myfloridalegal.com/webfiles.nsf/WF/JMEE-9AKRP2/%24file/
HHSLetter.pdf.

StateReforum. 2014. "State Approaches to Consumer Assistance Training." Updated March 6, 2014. Accessed March 8, 2015. https://www
.statereforum.org/consumer-assistance-training.

6

❖

The Health Care Industry and the Affordable Care Act

By 2022, health care spending is projected to account for nearly 20 percent of the United States' Gross Domestic Product (GDP)—a staggering number (Centers for Medicare and Medicaid Services, 2014). With so much of the nation's economic activity tied to health care, all changes large and small impact the health industry sectors in some way. The ACA is arguably the largest overhaul of the health system in our country's history—and its impacts on industry, including insurers, providers, and pharmaceutical and device manufacturers, have been complex. This chapter focuses on myths and claims about the law centered on the health care industry. In some cases there are legitimate debates on how the law is affecting industry, but in other cases technical provisions, such provisions aimed at stabilizing the new exchange markets for insurers, have been politicized and painted as "industry bailouts." The success of these policies is still open to debate (and subject to continuing politics), but one thing is certain—parts of the ACA were designed to change market conditions and incentives various parts of the health care industry operated under.

The broadest—and one of the most pervasive—myths about the law alleges that it is a government takeover of health care. Republicans and conservative policy experts have led much of their opposition to the law with this claim, as reflected in the writing of one conservative think tank: "The 2,700-page Patient Protection and Affordable Care Act created the architecture for the government-controlled health care system that the administration is busily constructing through thousands of pages of regulation" (Galen Institute, 2012). The claim reflects a general stance that the ACA's approach to solving the problems of rising numbers of uninsured Americans and unsustainable costs relies too heavily on government regulation—and not enough on the private sector and health care market forces.

Other myths and claims related to the private sector have also proliferated, with some directed at individual industries. For instance, reforms aimed at shifting the Medicare program from one that pays for volume of services delivered to one that pays for value realigned the financial incentives providers operated under. One mechanism for accomplishing this realignment is Accountable Care Organizations (ACOs) that hold providers jointly accountable for costs and quality of care provided to a population—and many proponents of ACOs claim that they will successfully improve care and contain costs in the long term. Other claims have focused on the health insurance industry—such as whether or not the ACA actually increases competition among insurers as it set out to do.

Q29. DOES THE AFFORDABLE CARE ACT AMOUNT TO A GOVERNMENT "TAKEOVER" OF THE AMERICAN HEALTH CARE SYSTEM?

Answer: No. In 2010, in fact, the Pulitzer Prize–winning Politifact.com, an independent fact-checking journalism website, called the charge that Obamacare was in effect a "government takeover of health care" their "Lie of the Year" (Adair and Holan, 2010).

The ACA does make a number of foundational changes to the health care system, namely by expanding coverage to a large proportion of the uninsured and by trying to move the health care system to one that pays for value over volume. However, it has largely done so by maintaining—or expanding—the reach of the private sector in providing coverage and care. Overall, the ACA has increased regulation over industry but has also maintained industry's role in designing, innovating, and delivering health care services and treatments.

The Facts: One of the most pervasive claims about the ACA is that it signals a government takeover of health care in the United States. The claim originated in the spring of 2009, very early in the health reform debate. As it became clear that the Democratic-controlled White House and Congress would undertake the massive efforts, Republicans worked to articulate their opposing positions. The origin of this claim can be tied to the work of a prominent Republican strategist, Frank Luntz. He crafted a defining memo for Republican Congressional leaders with recommendations on powerful communications and messages for outlining opposition to health reform, including that Republicans refer to health reform as a "government takeover" (Luntz, 2009). The memo gave birth to perhaps the most pervasive claim or myth about the ACA that continues to be repeated by ACA opponents and believed by large segments of the public.

Luntz's 28-page memo was titled "The Language of Health Care 2009: The 10 rules for stopping the 'Washington Takeover' of Health care." It gave Republicans recommendations on how to message and frame opposition to health reform to the general public. In the memo Luntz stresses the importance of using the words "government takeover" to describe health reform:

> "Time" is the government health care killer. . . . Nothing else turns people against the government takeover of health care than the realistic expectation that it will result in delayed and potentially even denied treatment, procedures and/or medications. . . . Delayed care is denied care. . . . You'll notice we recommend the phrase "government takeover" rather than "government run" or "government controlled" It's because too many politician say "we don't want a government run health care system like Canada or Great Britain" without explaining those consequences. There is a better approach. "In countries with government run health care, politicians make YOUR health care decisions. THEY decide if you'll get the procedure you need, or if you are disqualified because the treatment is too expensive or because you are too old. We can't have that in America." (Luntz, 2009)

The memo was critical in shaping the debate early on—with much of the terminology and attack lines Luntz formulated against health reform taking firm root.

But the Luntz memo does not accurately represent the law and its provisions. The ACA has made structural changes to the health care industry in the United States and has led to new requirements and regulations on health plans, providers, and the pharmaceutical and device industry, but the government has not taken over any industry or the health care system at large (Adair and Holan, 2010). While there was discussion during the health reform debate about the inclusion of a government-run health plan to operate in the insurance exchanges—called the public plan—in the end it was not included in the law. It proved to be one of the most controversial provisions even among Democrats as it would have established a government-run health insurance plan to compete alongside commercial plans in the exchanges. In particular, conservative and moderate Democrats in the Senate, such as Sen. Joseph Lieberman (I-CT), were strongly opposed to the idea of a public plan. In the end, a public option was not included in the ACA—and so the insurance plans in the exchanges are all commercial or private in nature, as are providers that deliver care, and the pharmaceutical and device sector. When the ACA is actually examined, there is little evidence that the government is running the health care system.

However, if you examine the main components of the ACA, there is no evidence that the government is taking over the health care system—only that there is greater regulation over the industry to create a more equitable insurance market that increases the numbers of Americans with insurance and access to health care services, and to try to make the system more fiscally sustainable over time. The simplest explanation for why the ACA is not a government takeover of health care is that all health care industries remain private. For instance, 149 million Americans receive private coverage through their employers, ensuring that this channel continues to be the backbone of health insurance provision in the United States (Henry J. Kaiser Family Foundation and Health Research & Educational Trust, 2014). Providers (e.g., physicians, hospitals, and other facilities) remain private and are not owned or operated by the government. Life sciences companies that produce pharmaceutical and medical device products also remain private companies. Most important, the up to 24 million Americans projected to enroll in coverage through the ACA's health insurance exchanges will have access to only private or commercial insurance options (Congressional Budget Office, 2015). However, during the health reform debate in 2009, there was considerable controversy over a provision—the public option—that would have extended the government's reach into the private health insurance market, although it was never included in the final law.

While the federal government provides publicly funded health insurance through a number of programs, the most prominent of which are Medicare, Medicaid, and the Children's Health Insurance Program, a public option as part of health reform would have been distinct from existing government-operated sources of insurance. The public option would have established a government-run health insurance plan that would have operated alongside private, commercial plans in the exchanges. Progressive

Democrats largely supported the provision; however, many moderate and conservative Democrats and republicans were opposed. Officially, the White House supported the inclusion of a public option, stating in public materials that it was critical to reducing health care costs:

> Health reform must be built on three fundamental principles: It must lower the skyrocketing cost of health care; guarantee choice of doctors and plans; and assure quality affordable health care for every American. A public option would achieve those goals and give the American people more choices. It would foster greater competition; lower costs; and give consumers a greater variety of affordable choices. (The White House, 2010)

Throughout the health reform debate, especially in the Senate, the public option proved to be one of the most contentious issues—even among Democrats. Progressive Democrats supported the inclusion of a government-run health insurance option that would operate alongside private, commercial insurance in the health insurance exchanges. In the House legislation, the Congressional Budget Office projected that 20 percent of all exchange consumers would enroll in the public option (Congressional Budget Office, 2009). In the Senate, support for a public option was less solid and its inclusion in a final health reform bill was debated right up until the ACA's passage in the chamber in December 2009. Along the way, there were several attempts at compromises between Senate Democrats (and Republicans when bipartisan negotiations were still under way). The most prominent attempt was Sen. Kent Conrad's (D-ND) Consumer Oriented and Operated Plan (CO-OP). He introduced the idea early in a closed-door bipartisan meeting of senior members of the Finance and Help Committees in late spring 2009. The proposal was intended to be a compromise on the public plan. The CO-Ops would operate as nonprofit health insurance plans that would abide by the same rules as the private plans in the exchanges, but serve as an alternative to traditional commercial insurers for consumers. Senator Conrad's (D-ND) policy solution was aimed at solving one of the most divisive political problems in the debate:

> The strength of this proposal is that it accomplishes much of what those who want a public option are calling for—that is, something to compete with private for-profit insurance companies. . . . On the other hand, it meets the objections of many Republicans and some Democrats as well. The co-op is not government-controlled. (Volsky, 2009)

The CO-OPs remained in the final version of the ACA that was signed into law, but they were never fully accepted by both sides as a compromise. In the fall of 2009, as the Senate began its floor debate on health reform, proponents of the public option continued to push for its inclusion in the final legislation. However, conservative and moderate Democrats were opposed. One of the most prominent was Sen. Joseph Lieberman (I-CT), who was Independent, but caucused with the Democrats. He threatened to help filibuster health reform if a public option was included, stating:

> We're trying to do too much at once. . . . To put this government-created insurance company on top of everything else is just asking for trouble for the taxpayers, for the premium payers and for the national debt. I don't think we need it now. (Raju, 2009)

For health reform to pass the Senate, 60 votes were necessary to avoid a filibuster—which meant that every Democratic vote would be needed—or nearly every vote would be needed if Senator Olympia Snowe (R-ME) were convinced to vote for the final Senate version, which she did not. To keep most Democratic votes together and to woo Senator Snowe, the public plan was not included in the ACA. As a whole, the ACA keeps the private health care system in the United States intact; while there is greater regulation and new requirements across the industry, the law leverages private insurance companies, private providers, and life sciences companies to expand access to insurance, and health care services, treatments, and products.

FURTHER READING

Adair, B., and Holan, A. 2010. "Politifact's Lie of the Year: 'A government takeover of health care.'" Politifact.com. December 16, 2010. Accessed March 14, 2015. http://www.politifact.com/truth-o-meter/article/2010/dec/16/lie-year-government-takeover-health-care/.

Centers for Medicare and Medicaid Services. 2014. "Table 1. National Health Expenditures; Aggregate and Per Capita Amounts, Annual Percent Change and Percent Distribution: Selected Calendar Years 1960–2012." Accessed April 26, 2014. http://www.cms.gov/Research-Statistics-Data-and-Systems/Statistics-Trends-and-Reports/NationalHealthExpendData/Downloads/Proj2012.pdf.

Congressional Budget Office. 2015. "Insurance Coverage Provisions of the Affordable Care Act—CBO's March 2015 Baseline." Accessed March 10, 2015. http://www.cbo.gov/sites/default/files/cbofiles/attachments/43900-2015-03-ACAtables.pdf.

Congressional Budget Office. 2009. "Letter to the Honorable Charles B. Rangel. October 29, 2009." Accessed October 8, 2015. http://www .cbo.gov/sites/default/files/111th-congress-2009-2010/costestimate/ hr3962rangel0.pdf.

Galen Institute. 2012. "10 Reasons ObamaCare Is a Government Take-over of Health Care." Fall 2012. Accessed April 27, 2015. http://www .galen.org/assets/02-govt-takeover1.pdf.

Henry J. Kaiser Family Foundation & Health Research Educational Trust. 2014. "Employer Health Benefits: 2014 Annual Survey." Accessed January 3, 2015. http://files.kff.org/attachment/2014-employer-heal th-benefits-survey-full-report.

Luntz, F. 2009. "The Language of Health Care 2009: The 10 Rules for Stopping the 'Washington Takeover' of Health Care." Accessed March 11, 2015. http://www.politico.com/static/PPM116_luntz.html.

Raju, M. 2009. "Joe Lieberman: I'll Block Vote on Harry Reid's Plan." Polit-ico. October 27, 2009. Accessed March 14, 2015. http://www.politico .com/news/stories/1009/28788.html.

Volsky, I. 2009. "Conrad Proposes Co-ops to Replace Public Plan." Think Progress. June 10, 2009. Accessed March 14, 2015. http://thinkprog ress.org/health/2009/06/10/170816/conrad-coop/.

The White House. 2010. "Health Insurance Reform Reality Check." Accessed March 14, 2015. https://www.whitehouse.gov/realitycheck/faq#i2.

Q30. WILL ACCOUNTABLE CARE ORGANIZATIONS (ACOs) IMPROVE QUALITY AND REDUCE HEALTH CARE COSTS?

Answer: While the long-term impacts of ACOs are unknown, early results from ACO efforts have demonstrated promise in improving quality. Reducing costs has been more challenging and will likely take more time to demonstrate and to assess the impacts of ACOs in that regard.

The Facts: The term "accountable care organization" (ACO) was coined in 2006 by Dr. Elliott Fisher at a Medicare Payment Advisory Commission meeting (Fisher et al., 2007). Generally, ACOs hold a group of providers jointly accountable for the cost and quality of care delivered to a defined population. In a relatively short period, ACOs have gone from largely being a concept for how to change care delivery in the United States to being one of the most tested new models in the country with both public and private payers.

While the term ACO predates health reform, passage of the Affordable Care Act was a catalyst for the concept to take root across the country in response to growing costs and quality problems in the U.S. health care system. In particular, the ACA established the Medicare Shared Savings Program (MSSP), which allows providers to form ACOs. Participating providers are then held to specified quality and cost targets. If participating ACOs meet both the cost and quality targets, then they are eligible to share in any savings with the federal government. In addition to the MSSP, the Centers for Medicare and Medicaid Services (CMS) has begun operating other ACO programs to test different models and payment approaches. In 2015, CMS reported 404 Medicare ACOs across the country were serving over 7.3 million Medicare beneficiaries (Centers for Medicare and Medicaid Services, 2015). Spurred by this activity, commercial ACOs are also proliferating and solidifying its potential as a model for controlling costs and improving quality over the long term.

However, conservatives alleged that ACOs would not control costs but would lead to greater government control over health care and even possibly end in the creation of a single-payer system, which was strongly opposed by Republicans (Hoff, 2011; Johnson, 2010). One commentary published by the conservative Heritage Foundation stated:

> There is much to dislike about this year's massive federal overhaul of the nation's health care system. One of Obamacare's potentially most dangerous—and least discussed—features is its call for government-sponsored accountable care organizations (ACOs). (Johnson, 2010)

However, the proliferation of ACOs among both public and private payers, as well as providers, does not indicate that the model has led to greater government control or a single-payer system.

ACOs are physicians and other providers that agree to be jointly held accountable for the cost and quality of care a defined group of patients receives across settings and participating providers. Both private and public payers, including Medicare and Medicaid, are piloting programs across the country, underscoring how quickly ACOs have moved from an idea Dr. Fisher and others coined in 2007 to becoming one of the leading examples of change in the U.S. health care system today. Prior to the ACA, Medicare did not have the option for providers to form ACOs. However, the law established the MSSP, a voluntary demonstration in which participating providers form ACOs. ACOs that meet quality require-ments and reduce costs relative to projected benchmarks are then eligible to share in a percentage of the savings. In April 2015, CMS reported there were 404 Medicare ACOs across the country—a remarkable num-ber given that they were introduced to the Medicare program as recently as 2010 (Centers for Medicare and Medicaid Services, 2015). In addition to the MSSP, the ACA established the Center for Medicare and Medicaid Innovation (CMMI), which received $10 billion of funding over 10 years to test new payment and delivery models in health care that can reduce federal health care costs, while also improving quality. CMMI has also played a role in expanding ACO models through additional programs, such as the Pioneer and Next Generation programs that are expected to include approximately 40 advanced health care systems that can assume higher levels of risk compared to MSSP participants in being accountable for the costs and quality of care patients receive.

Following Medicare's lead, commercial payers are also experimenting heavily with ACOs in an effort to improve quality and control medical cost trend. Leavitt Partners, a health care consulting firm, estimates that there are over 250 commercial or private ACOs across the country (Muh-lestein, 2014).

In addition to private ACOs, Medicaid programs across the country have turned to the model as a way to address growing budget pressures and higher levels of enrollment into the program. Historically, Medicaid has been siloed relative to other payers; however, the imperative to control costs and quality has led to new cross-payer initiatives, leading Medicaid to experiment in ways the program has not done in the past. By one esti-mate, 18 states are actively forming ACOs in some capacity (Maxwell et al., 2014).

While Medicaid has been slower to develop ACOs relative to Medicare or commercial payers, the safety net program's move toward the model underscores how widespread it is becoming. Finally, an important metric for how widespread the ACO model is, according to one expert, is to estimate the number of lives served by ACO arrangements, which could be as high as 18 million lives across public and private payers—or approx-imately 5 percent of the U.S. population (Muhlestein, 2014). Clearly, ACOs have taken hold among a diversity of payers and are changing care delivery for a measurable percentage of the U.S. population.

Despite the model's popularity and early promise, there are still a number of detractors. The Heritage Foundation published a number of opinion pieces on the negative impacts ACOs would have on American health care. Much of the criticism alleges that ACOs will lead to greater government control over health care:

> Among the power elite in Washington, ACOs have great appeal as a mechanism through which they can exercise benevolent control. The unspoken premise of Obamacare is that government officials know far better than we do what is good for us. In their heart of hearts, most Obamacare proponents probably prefer a single-payer system. ACOs may be used as a cornerstone for building just such a system. (Johnson, 2010)

Other opinion pieces echoed the charge that ACOs are first and foremost a tool for the government to exercise greater control over individual's health care choices (Hoff, 2011). However, if ACOs were another mechanism for facilitating government control over health care, private-sector interest by both payer and providers would not likely be as robust. For instance, national insurers, such as Aetna and Cigna have made significant investments in creating ACOs or at least using accountable care principles to improve quality and control costs (Accountable Care Solutions, 2015; Cigna, 2015). For instance, Cigna reports having 122 accountable care arrangements with large physician groups in 29 states, serving 1.3 million lives (Cigna, 2015).

ACO criticisms have also centered on the actual design features of ACOs, such as:

- inability to engage patients in their own care;
- lack of provider accountability by maintaining or building on existing fee-for-service system;
- driving provider consolidation due to health information technology and other infrastructure needs (Numerof, 2011).

ACOs have come under a wide range of criticisms, but the more valid ones focus on how the payment and care delivery design features will impact quality of care, patient outcomes and experience, and cost; however, initial results suggest that ACOs are achieving some of the goals they set out to.

Early results indicate that ACOs can improve outcomes but that cost reduction is more difficult. Results from the second year of the MSSP ACO program indicated that ACOs showed improvement on nearly all quality and patient experience measures—so it appears that the new delivery mechanism can positively impact patient care and experience (Centers for Medicare and Medicaid Services, 2014a). Approximately half of the year two participants also reduced costs relative to their spending benchmarks; however, only 25 percent reduced costs enough to earn shared savings (Centers for Medicare and Medicaid Services, 2014b). So while nearly all participants improved quality and patient experience, not all were able to reduce costs—especially enough to earn shared savings. Private-sector ACOs are also reporting early results, such as Cigna's Collaborative Care program, which reported that 74 percent of those in the program for two or more years had both 2 percent better cost and quality performance relative to the broader market (Cigna, 2015).

ACOs are not a silver bullet for the U.S. health care system's cost and quality challenges; however, the goals they espouse—to foster greater accountability for the quality and cost of patient care across providers and settings—are part of a greater movement in the system to pay for value over volume. At a minimum, ACOs are connecting providers across setting, focusing on patient outcomes and experience as critical goals in care, and trying to reduce costs by holding providers accountable for a patient's total cost of care.

FURTHER READING

Accountable Care Solutions. 2015. "Accountable Care Solutions from Aetna." Accessed May 26, 2015. http://www.aetnaacs.com/what-accountable-care.

Centers for Medicare and Medicaid Services. 2014a. "Fact Sheets: Medicare ACOs Continue to Succeed in Improving Care, Lowering Cost Growth." Accessed March 21, 2015. http://www.cms.gov/Newsroom/MediaReleaseDatabase/Fact-sheets/2014-Fact-sheets-items/2014-09-16.html.

Centers for Medicare and Medicaid Services. 2014b. "Medicare ACOs Continue to Succeed in Improving Care, Lowering Cost Growth." Accessed March 14, 2015. http://www.cms.gov/Newsroom/MediaReleaseDatabase/Fact-sheets/2014-Fact-sheets-items/2014-11-10.html.

Centers for Medicare and Medicaid Services. 2015. "Fast Facts—All Medicare Shared Savings Program ACOs." Accessed May 26, 2015. http://www.cms.gov/Medicare/Medicare-Fee-for-Service-Payment/sharedsavingsprogram/Downloads/All-Starts-MSSP-ACO.pdf.

Cigna. 2015. "Cigna Collaborative Care." Accessed March 21, 2015. http://newsroom.cigna.com/knowledgecenter/aco.

Fisher, E., Staiger, D., Bynum, J., and Gottlieb, D. 2007. "Creating accountable care organizations: The extended hospital medical staff." *Health Affairs*, 26, 1: w44–w57.

Hoff, J. 2011. "Accountable Care Organization: Obamacare's Magic Bullet Misfires." The Heritage Foundation. Accessed March 17, 2015.

http://www.heritage.org/research/reports/2011/08/accountable-car
e-organizations-obamacares-magic-bullet-misfires.

Johnson, D. 2010. "Patient Beware of Accountable Care Organization."
The Heritage Foundation. Accessed March 14, 2015. http://www.her
itage.org/research/commentary/2010/10/patient-beware-of-accountabl
e-care-organization.

Maxwell, J., Bailit, M., Tobey, R., and Barron, C. 2014. "Early Observa-
tions Show Safety-Net ACOs Hold Promise to Achieve the Triple Aim
and Promote Health Equity." http://healthaffairs.org/blog/2014/09/15/
early-observations-show-safety-net-acos-hold-promise-to-achieve-
the-triple-aim-and-promote-health-equity/.

Muhlestein, D. 2014. "Accountable Care Growth in 2014: A Look Ahead."
Health Affairs Blog. Accessed March 20, 2015. http://healthaffairs.org/
blog/2014/01/29/accountable-care-growth-in-2014-a-look-ahead/.

Numerof, R. 2011. "Why Accountable Care Organizations Won't Deliver
Better Health Care—and Market Innovation Will." The Heritage Foundation. Accessed March 14, 2015. http://www.heritage.org/research/
reports/2011/04/why-accountable-care-organizations-wont-deliver-
better-health-care-and-market-innovation-will.

Q31. DID THE AFFORDABLE CARE ACT "BAIL OUT" INSURANCE COMPANIES?

Answer: No, although the law does provide a financial safety net of sorts
to insurers in the event that medical costs for enrollees exceed expectations. ACA provisions added millions of customers to the insurance
industry, but a considerable number of these customers, such as people
with preexisting conditions, could have high medical costs that are difficult to predict in a new insurance market. At the same time, the law also
contained a variety of measures designed to limit premium increases and
cap industry profits.

The Facts: The ACA insurance market reforms that went into effect
in 2014, including ones prohibiting coverage denials based on preexisting
conditions, guaranteed issue, and limiting premium rating variations, are
intended to increase access to coverage for those with preexisting conditions. Coupled with the insurance market reforms, the ACA provides
premium subsidies to individuals for whom insurance may have been previously unaffordable. These changes (among others) have made it difficult for insurers to predict who will enroll in coverage—especially in

the first few years of the ACA's health insurance exchanges—and what their resulting medical costs may be. Predicting medical costs is critical to ensuring premiums charged to enrollees are sufficient to cover the group's medical costs.

To protect against the uncertainty in the risk in the health insurance exchange markets, the ACA included three mechanisms—risk corridors, reinsurance, and risk adjustment—collectively known as the 3Rs. The first two are in effect from 2014 through 2016, and risk adjustment continues in perpetuity. Each of the mechanisms is designed to mitigate the uncertainty insurers face in the new markets, while also reducing any incentive they have to select risk (i.e., finding ways through benefit design or other mechanisms to attract healthier enrollees into their plans).

One of the primary goals of the ACA was to expand access to health insurance coverage to the nearly 50 million Americans who were uninsured at the time of the law's passage (DeNavas, Proctor, and Smith, 2011). Two of the primary mechanisms for expanding coverage were the passage of new insurance market reforms and premium subsidies to offset the cost of coverage for millions of Americans. First, starting in 2014 insurers were prohibited from denying coverage to individuals based on preexisting conditions, and were subject to guaranteed issue—ensuring anyone who wanted to purchase coverage could. Second, the law also prohibited insurers from varying health insurance premiums based on health status or gender (but did allow for limited variation based on other factors such as age). These changes made it more likely that individuals with preexisting conditions—and unmet health needs—would enroll in coverage when the health insurance exchanges launched in 2014. In addition, the new premium subsidies that would be offered to individuals and families with incomes from 100 to 400 percent of the Federal Poverty Level would make insurance much more affordable for many low- and middle-income Americans. Coupled together, these changes addressed two main barriers to purchasing insurance—the presence of preexisting conditions and affordability; but they also created an uncertain risk pool for insurers considering operating in the new exchanges in the initial years after their launch.

Mechanisms to mitigate the risk that insurers and providers face in covering and providing care through many different health care programs and plans are commonplace—especially when new programs launch and there is uncertainty about the health needs and profiles of those enrolling. For instance, when the Medicare Part D drug benefit launched, all seniors gained access to prescription drug coverage through Medicare for the first time. To stabilize the market, and mitigate the risk insurers faced in pricing accurate premiums for the new benefit, lawmakers included the same risk mitigation mechanisms in Medicare Part D as in the ACA—risk corridors, reinsurance, and risk adjustment. Medicare Part D received bipartisan support in Congress, underscoring that these are well-accepted mechanisms for stabilizing markets—and attracting insurers to participate in new markets.

First, risk adjustment is a mechanism in the ACA that discourages insurers from selecting risk (i.e., healthier individuals) to reduce their medical costs by transferring payments from insurers with lower-risk enrollees to those with higher-risk or sicker enrollees (Henry J. Kaiser Family Foundation, 2014). The program is budget neutral because it redistributes payments across insurers. Second, the ACA included a reinsurance program to stabilize premiums in the reformed individual market—and reduce plans' incentives to charge high premiums to account for individuals with high-cost medical needs enrolling in plans. The program was authorized for the first three years of the insurance exchanges through 2016, when most new enrollees would be expected and plans would have the most difficulty predicting the medical costs and risks they could assume. The ACA's reinsurance programs requires all private health plans, including employer-sponsored plans, to contribute $63 per person in 2014 and $44 per person in 2015 to the program (Henry J. Kaiser Family Foundation, 2014). In total, the program collected $10 billion in funds for 2014 and $6 billion for 2015 and is projected to collect $4 billion for 2016, reflecting the reduced need for stabilizing premiums as insurers gain more experience with the new individual market risk pool (Henry J. Kaiser Family Foundation, 2014). The program's funds are then distributed to plans that enroll high-cost enrollees—defined as those with $45,000 in insurer costs in 2014 and $70,000 in 2015 (Henry J. Kaiser Family Foundation, 2014). Finally, risk corridors have been used to encourage plans to set accurate premiums—especially high premiums given the uncertainty of the enrollee risk pool. The program essentially collects funds from payers that overpriced premiums based on defined parameters, and distributes funds to payers that underpriced their premiums from 2014 through 2016. All three are well-accepted mechanisms for stabilizing premiums—especially when establishing new markets and reducing risk selection by insurers.

The risk corridors program in particular has sparked significant controversy—mostly due to the mechanism by which it is funded. Unlike the other two programs, the risk corridor program is not expected to be budget neutral. So, if funds coming to the program from insurers were less than funds being paid out, the federal government would presumably cover the additional costs.

The lack of clarity about the backup funding for the risk corridors program was seized on by Obamacare critics, who described it as essentially a government bailout of insurance companies. This criticism intensified in the fall of 2013, when the Obama Administration announced that state plans that did not meet the new ACA requirements could still be sold temporarily. One of the most vocal critics of the program has been Sen. Marco Rubio (R-FL), who introduced legislation to repeal the risk corridor program (S.1726, 2013). His public statements underscored how this technical provision aimed at promoting accurate premium pricing in the ACA exchanges became political:

> One of the biggest threats to the American Dream is the rising cost of living, which ObamaCare is making worse through rising health care costs and loss of coverage. . . . Taxpayers should not have to fund massive bailouts to protect the profits of the insurance companies that helped write Obamacare, which is why I've been fighting for over a year to protect taxpayers from yet another bailout that puts them on the hook for Washington's mistakes. (Rubio, 2013)

Rubio's legislation, the Obamacare Taxpayer Bailout Prevention Act, would have repealed the risk corridors provision altogether. The logic underpinning Rubio's bill was that the program was not budget neutral and that the federal government would have to make funds available if plans systematically underpriced their products to attract enrollees. There was little to no bipartisan support for such a policy, especially given that the exchanges were about to launch and insurers were facing a great deal of uncertainty about the enrollees in the new market.

A closer look at the structure of the 3Rs programs, as well as their impact on the initial impact they have had on the health insurance exchanges, suggests that they are having their intended impacts. When the final regulations on the 3Rs provisions were released, the Robert Wood Johnson Foundation and the Wakely Consulting Group released a nonpartisan issue brief analyzing the provisions. The authors conclude:

> While a number of important details are outstanding and some critical questions still remain, our opinion is that the final rules are logical and provide a good structure for these important programs. They allow states flexibility while still providing federal support. The programs provide significant financial protections which are necessary given the market and financial uncertainties created under the ACA. (Winkelman et al., 2012)

Examining health insurance exchange market trends from 2014 to 2015 also suggests that the risk adjustment, reinsurance, and risk corridor programs are functioning as envisioned. First, the Department of Health and Human Services (HHS) estimates that the number of insurers participating in the health insurance exchanges from 2014 to 2015 increased by 25 percent—a sizable number—suggesting that the marketplaces were viewed as relatively stable and attractive for competition (Gunja and Gee, 2014). Second, enrollment in the exchanges reached 11.7 million individuals by the end of the second open enrollment period (Assistant Secretary for Planning and Evaluation, 2015). The evidence suggests that the 3Rs programs are functioning as intending—by creating viable insurance exchanges for insurers to compete in to cover many individuals and families who formerly were unable to access coverage.

FURTHER READING

Assistant Secretary for Planning and Evaluation, 2015. "Health Insurance Marketplaces 2015 Open Enrollment Period: March Enrollment Report." Accessed March 22, 2015. http://aspe.hhs.gov/health/reports/2015/MarketPlaceEnrollment/Mar2015/ib_2015mar_enrollment.pdf.

DeNavas, C., Proctor, B., and Smith, J. 2011. "Income, Poverty, and Health Insurance Coverage in the United States: 2010." United States Census Bureau. Accessed February 28, 2015. http://www.census.gov/prod/2011pubs/p60-239.pdf.

Gunja, M., and Gee, E. 2014. "Health Insurance Issuer Participation and New Entrants in the Health Insurance Marketplace in 2015." Assistant Secretary for Planning and Evaluation. Accessed March 22, 2015. http://aspe.hhs.gov/health/reports/2014/NewEntrants/ib_NewEntrants.pdf.

Henry J. Kaiser Family Foundation. 2014. "Explaining Health Care Reform: Risk Adjustment, Reinsurance, and Risk Corridors." Accessed March 22, 2015. http://kff.org/health-reform/issue-brief/explaining-health-care-reform-risk-adjustment-reinsurance-and-risk-corridors/.

Rubio, M. 2013. "Rubio Introduces Bill Preventing Taxpayer-Funded Bailouts of Insurance Companies under Obamacare." Accessed March 22, 2015. http://www.rubio.senate.gov/public/index.cfm/press-releases?ID=fc464be2-7d88-4157-b6c1-aad18595e81c.

S. 1726. 2013. "Obamacare Taxpayer Bailout Prevention Act." Accessed March 21, 2015. https://www.congress.gov/bill/113th-congress/senate-bill/1726.

Winkelman, R., Peper, J., Holland, P., Mehmud, S., and Woolman, J. 2012. "Analysis of HHS Final Rules on Reinsurance, Risk Corridors and Risk Adjustment." Robert Wood Johnson Foundation. Accessed March 22, 2015. http://www.rwjf.org/content/dam/farm/reports/issue_briefs/2012/rwjf72568.

Q32. WILL THE AFFORDABLE CARE ACT INCREASE MARKET COMPETITION AMONG INSURERS?

Answer: Early indications are that the ACA was increasing competition among health insurers, which was a major goal of the law's architects. In general, the majority of studies done on market competition in the exchanges from 2014 to 2015 indicate that more insurers are entering the health insurance exchanges than before and that the new markets are functioning as envisioned. However, future competitiveness could be undermined by proposed mergers among the largest insurers in the country.

The Facts: Prior to the ACA, insurance markets in many states were often dominated by a single insurer. One analysis found that in 30 states and the District of Columbia, a single insurer controlled half of the individual market in 2010 (Henry J. Kaiser Family Foundation, 2011). This lack of competition has been regarded as one of the reasons that premium prices were unaffordable—and steadily increasing leading to nearly 50 million Americans being uninsured in 2010 when the ACA passed (DeNavas, Proctor, and Smith, 2011). One of the impacts of the ACA's health insurance exchanges was to create regulated markets where multiple plans would compete on cost—and not risk selection.

In response to this market consolidation, the ACA's insurance exchanges were intended to stimulate greater competition by encouraging insurers to enter these new markets and compete to cover the influx of projected new lives. In turn, the addition competition would provide consumers with greater choice and help constrain premium prices.

This concept of "managed competition" first gained widespread notice in the early 1990s during the Clinton health reform effort. Dr. Alain Enthoven developed the idea through the 1970s and into the 1990s when the term became more widely understood and used (Enthoven, 2014). There were three main components of Enthoven's theory for how costs would be constrained: (1) provision of comprehensives of services and benefits, (2) individual choice to switch plans, and (3) "sponsors" or "market organizers" that "enforce principles of equity," such as guaranteed issue, subsidized access to lowest cost plans, and premium rating rules (Enthoven, 1993). Nearly 20 years later, managed competition informed the creation of the ACA exchanges, with the hopes that they would spur greater competition among plans.

In 2011, the Henry J. Kaiser Family Foundation released a study on competition in insurance markets using a variety of data sources, including the percentage of people in a market enrolled by a single insurer in a state, the number of insurance carriers in a market, and a measure of how evenly market share is spread across insurers (Henry J. Kaiser Family Foundation, 2011). The study found the individual market was "highly concentrated" in many states, with 30 states and the District of Columbia having a single insurance company with over 50 percent market share (Henry J. Kaiser Family Foundation, 2011).

Clearly, there is variability across the United States, but one-third of all states had one insurer controlling over 65 percent of the market, with single insurers in Alabama and Iowa controlling 86 and 84 percent of the market, respectively (Henry J. Kaiser Family Foundation, 2011). The Government Accountability Office has also been studying market competition, as required by the ACA. Their baseline analysis released in 2013 before the exchanges and insurance market reforms went into effect found that across a state's individual, small-group, and large-group markets, enrollment was concentrated in the three largest insurers in the state (Government Accountability Office, 2014).

The goal to increase consumer choice—and thus spur price competition that would make policies more affordable—emerged as a major Democratic point of emphasis in the health reform debate. In 2009, President Obama stated in a speech to Congress:

> Now, if you're one of the tens of millions of Americans who don't currently have health insurance, the second part of this plan will finally offer you quality, affordable choices. If you lose your job or you change your job, you'll be able to get coverage. If you strike out on your own and start a small business, you'll be able to get coverage. We'll do this by creating a new insurance exchange—a marketplace where individuals and small businesses will be able to shop for health insurance at competitive prices. Insurance companies will have an incentive to participate in this exchange because it lets them compete for millions of new customers. As one big group, these customers will have greater leverage to bargain with the insurance companies for better prices and quality coverage. (The White House, 2009)

The ACA sought to spur competition and greater value among insurers by weakening the dominance of a small number of insurers at the national and state levels.

Conservative critics of the law did not believe the ACA would be successful in promoting competition among insurance plans. To the contrary, they predicted that the new coverage requirements and other regulations in the law would dampen insurer participation in the exchanges, lead to smaller insurers leaving the market, and limit the entry of new insurers (Haislmaier, 2013). An analysis by the conservative Heritage Foundation compared insurer participation in the exchanges with participation in the pre-ACA individual market, and concluded that insurer participation was 36 percent lower after the insurance exchanges launched (Singer, 2014).

On the other hand, a recent study of level of competition in seven states by the nonpartisan Henry J. Kaiser Family Foundation came to a more nuanced conclusion after examining individual state insurance markets in 2012 and again in 2014. They concluded that states such as California and New York were significantly more competitive after the ACA, but that Connecticut and Washington were less competitive because of insurers declining to participate in the exchanges (Cox et al., 2014).

It is difficult to come to any firm conclusion based on these early data; however, simply looking at the number of insurers is insufficient for a complete picture on insurer competition, as it provides information only on consumer choice and not competition.

A more accurate assessment of market competition as a result of the ACA may be to make comparisons based on multiple factors—including the number of insurers participating, choice of carriers, and percent market share starting from 2014 onward. On the first point, HHS estimates there was a 25 percent increase in new issuers entering the exchanges from 2014 to 2015 (Gunja and Gee, 2014). One of the primary signs that the exchange markets were viewed as viable and as promising business opportunities was the greater participation of large, national insurers—some of whom elected to limit participation in exchanges in 2014 (Gunja and Gee, 2014). For instance, large national insurers, such as Aetna, United Health care, and Cigna, limited their exchange participation in 2014 in the face of uncertainty about the risk profiles of those that would enroll (Luhby, 2013). Aetna, for instance, pulled out of one-third of the states it initially planned to participate in (Luhby, 2013). However, in 2015 all three expanded the number of exchanges they participated in (Japsen, 2014). The business decision these large national insurers have made to enter more individual exchange markets suggests they believe the markets are viable and offer opportunities to expand their current market shares.

In addition, one goal of increasing insurer participation in the exchanges is to allow choice to drive price competition. The nonpartisan McKinsey Center for U.S. Health Reform concluded that competition and choice in the exchanges were increasing as health insurer participation increased in 2015, and the number of products—especially in the silver tier that subsidies are tied to—also increased (McKinsey Center for U.S. Health System Reform, 2014). The markers of whether the individual market is more competitive after the ACA require multiple data points—and not just the number of insurers or carriers in a market—and the impacts across states will vary widely depending on history, insurer participation, population size, and other factors. In addition, proposed mergers between some of the largest insurers in the country, such as Aetna and Humana and Anthem and Cigna, could change competition in the exchanges moving forward. A more conclusive assessment of how the ACA has impacted insurance market competition will also be more possible starting in 2017 when the reinsurance and risk corridors mechanisms to stabilize the market and incent insurer participation in the exchanges have ended. However, at a minimum, the ACA has led to more comparable insurance plans across issuers and appears to be leading to more competitive exchanges in the first few years of implementation as well.

FURTHER READING

Cox, C., Levitt, L., Claxton, G., Ma, R., and Duddy-Tenbrunsel, R. 2015. "Analysis of 2015 Premium Changes in the Affordable Care Act's Health Insurance Marketplaces." Henry J. Kaiser Family Foundation. Accessed February 25, 2015. http://files.kff.org/attachment/analysis-of-2015-premium-changes-in-the-affordable-care-acts-health-insurance-marketplaces-issue-brief.

Cox, C., Ma, R., Claxton, G., and Levitt, L. 2014. "Sizing Up Exchange Market Competition." Henry J. Kaiser Family Foundation. Accessed March 25, 2015. http://kff.org/health-reform/issue-brief/sizing-up-exchange-market-competition/.

DeNavas, C., Proctor, B., and Smith, J. 2011. "Income, Poverty, and Health Insurance Coverage in the United States: 2010." United States Census Bureau. Accessed February 28, 2015. http://www.census.gov/prod/2011pubs/p60-239.pdf.

Enthoven, A. 1993. "The History and Principles of Managed Competition." *Health Affairs*, Supplement 1993. Accessed March 25, 2015. http://content.healthaffairs.org/content/12/suppl_1/24.full.pdf+html.

Enthoven, A. 2014. "Managed Competition by the Private Sector: Rescued by the Private Sector?" *Health Affairs Blog*. Accessed March 25,

2015. http://healthaffairs.org/blog/2014/05/12/managed-competition-2014-rescued-by-the-private-sector/.

Government Accountability Office. 2014. "Private Health Insurance: Concentration of Enrollees among Individual, Small Group, and Large Group Insurers from 2010 through 2013." Accessed March 25, 2015. http://www.gao.gov/assets/670/667245.pdf.

Gunja, M., and Gee, E. 2014. "Health Insurance Issuer Participation and New Entrants in the Health Insurance Marketplace in 2015." Assistant Secretary for Planning and Evaluation. Accessed March 25, 2015. http://aspe.hhs.gov/health/reports/2014/NewEntrants/ib_NewEntrants.pdf.

Haislmaier, E. 2013. "Health Insurers' Decisions on Exchange Participation: Obamacare's Leading Indicators." The Heritage Foundation. Accessed March 25, 2015. http://www.heritage.org/research/reports/2013/11/health-insurers-decisions-on-exchange-participation-obamacares-leading-indicators.

Henry J. Kaiser Family Foundation. 2011. "How Competitive Are State Insurance Markets?" Accessed March 23, 2015. https://kaiserfamily foundation.files.wordpress.com/2013/01/8242.pdf.

Japsen, B. 2014. "Cigna to Expand on Obamacare Exchanges in 2015." Forbes. July 31, 2014. Accessed March 25, 2015. http://www.forbes.com/sites/brucejapsen/2014/07/31/cigna-to-expand-on-obamacare-exchanges-in-2015/.

Luhby, T. 2013. "Big Insurers Ditch Obamacare Exchanges." Accessed March 25, 2015. *CNN Money*, November 10, 2013. Accessed March 25, 2015. http://money.cnn.com/2013/09/10/news/economy/obamacare-insurers/.

McKinsey Center for U.S. Health System Reform. 2014. "2015 OEP: Emerging Trends in the Individual Exchanges." McKinsey & Company. Accessed March 24, 2015. http://healthcare.mckinsey.com/open-enroll ment-emerging-trends.

Singer, A. 2014. "Measuring Choice and Competition in the Exchanges: Still Worse Than before the ACA." The Heritage Foundation. Accessed March 24, 2015. http://www.heritage.org/research/reports/2014/12/measuring-choice-and-competition-in-the-exchanges-still-worse-than-before-the-aca#_ftn1.

The White House. 2009. "Remarks by the President to a Joint Session of Congress on Health Care." Office of the Press Secretary. Accessed May 26, 2015. https://www.whitehouse.gov/the_press_office/Remarks-by-the-President-to-a-Joint-Session-of-Congress-on-Health-Care/.

7

❖❖❖

Individual and Community Health and the Affordable Care Act

While one of the main goals of health reform was to increase health insurance coverage for the uninsured, a primary reason for increasing access to insurance (and routine access to health care services as a result) is to improve individual health outcomes, as well as the health status of populations. This chapter reviews a number of myths and claims about the ACA related to individuals' access to health care providers and services, including preventive services at a community level. Unsurprisingly, these topics have generated significant controversy. For the most part, Democrats have claimed that law provides greater access to preventive care, that it strengthens primary care, and that it improves the health of individuals and communities through increased insurance coverage and new funding aimed at improving public health. On the other hand, Republicans have claimed that the changes in the ACA will actually reduce access to care by increasing wait times for those with insurance to see their providers as demand for health care services grows and provider shortages grow larger—leading to worse health outcomes and even rationing overseen by government entities with new authorities under the ACA.

There were two particularly controversial myths and claims about the ACA on how the law impacts individual and community health outcomes. First, the law established and funded the Prevention and Public Health Fund to make new investments in public health that would improve health outcomes and status. However, the open-ended nature of the funding and its uses came under fire from Republicans, who were successful in scaling the Fund back as a result. Second, the coverage requirements for effective preventive services increased accessibility to contraception for those with employer-sponsored insurance; however, private companies with religious objections to subsidizing contraceptive coverage led a legal challenge to the mandate—going all the way to the Supreme Court.

Q33. IS THE AFFORDABLE CARE ACT'S PREVENTION AND PUBLIC HEALTH FUND A "SLUSH FUND"?

Answer: Broadly, this fund has been used as intended, to supplement existing public health and prevention efforts aimed at improving the health of Americans and reducing health care costs. However, the Fund has been used in some cases to fill funding gaps for public health programs that have been subject to Republican budget cuts, so the conservative complaint that the Fund is being used to circumvent Congress does have some validity. And even some Democrats questioned the diversion of money in this Fund to aid in the rollout of the ACA's health insurance marketplaces.

The Facts: Title IV of the ACA, "Prevention of Chronic Disease and Improving Public Health," focused on prevention and public health issues. The title included a number of new programs, as well as funding for the efforts—the centerpiece of which was the Prevention and Public Health Trust Fund (the Fund). At the time of the ACA's passage, the Trust Fund was appropriated $15 billion over 10 years for "expanded and sustained national investments in public health, to improve health outcomes, and to enhance care quality" (Department of Health and Human Services, 2015). Since 2010, the Fund has been used for a wide array of activities, both within and outside the bounds of Congressional intent. For instance, it has been used to fund community and clinical prevention initiatives, to build public health infrastructure, and for tobacco prevention; however, it has also been used to fund the ACA's Navigator and consumer assister programs to help potential health insurance exchange enrollees—programs that may otherwise have had no funding (Department of Health and Human Services, 2015). The structure of the Fund, coupled with its funding level, made it a target for opponents of the law, who justified their attacks by calling it a "slush fund" for the Administration.

While there have been repeated attempts to repeal the Fund altogether in the House of Representatives, complete repeal has been unsuccessful and even faced a veto threat (Office of Management and Budget, 2011). However, the Fund has been one of the few parts of the ACA that Democrats and President Obama have agreed to reduce funding for in the course of budget negotiations. In 2012, budget negotiations resulted in an estimated $5 billion reduction in the Fund (H.R. 3630, 2012). The controversy and politicization of the fund have fueled attempts to repeal it altogether and have also allowed it to one of the few provisions in the ACA that has been scaled back.

The concept of the Prevention and Public Health Fund originated well before health reform. Its roots can be traced back to the Centers for Disease Control and Prevention's Prevention Block Grant, which dates back to 1986. In 2006, the Center for American Progress presented a more expansive version of the Prevention and Public Health Fund idea—a "Wellness Trust" that would include funding from existing Public Health Service grants and funding from Medicare, Medicaid, and other health programs (Lambrew and Podesta, 2006). Building on this idea, then senator Hillary Clinton (D-NY) introduced legislation to establish a Wellness Trust (S. 3674, 2008). As the Senate HELP Committee undertook health reform, Democratic Chairman Ted Kennedy (D-MA) charged Senator Tom Harkin (D-IA), a leader in the Senate on prevention issues, with spearheading the Committee's efforts on that front. Among other provisions, Senator Harkin, who would assume eventual Chairmanship of the HELP Committee, fought to establish the Prevention and Public Health Fund.

The ACA originally dedicated $15 billion to the Fund over an initial 10 years to invest in disease prevention and public health. In 2010, 7 of the top 10 causes of death in the United States were attributable to chronic diseases, and cancer and heart disease alone accounted for almost half of all deaths (Centers for Disease Control and Prevention, 2015). Chronic diseases also account for a disproportionate share of all health care spending, with estimates that 85 percent of all health care spending is due to chronic disease (Anderson, 2010). Coupled with these striking statistics that underscore the impact of chronic disease on mortality and health care costs, new studies emerged highlighting the benefits of prevention. For instance, the Trust for America's Health released a study in 2008 estimating that a $10 per person per year investment in effective community-based disease prevention could lead to a return on investment of $5.60 for every $1 spent within five years from medical cost savings (Trust for America's Health, 2008). These findings added to the momentum to make new investments in prevention and public health as part of health reform in such a way that allowed states and local governments to design or implement effective programs that responded to the unique health problems facing their communities. The Fund became central to a mission of health reform—to refocus the health system on population health outcomes in an effort to improve health and bend the cost curve.

The ongoing federal investment in the Fund was generally intended to supplement existing public health and prevention efforts and funding. However, the Fund has been used in many cases to fill funding gaps for public health programs that have been subject to budget cuts, as well as to promote the ACA's exchanges. For instance, most of the $500 million in funding in 2010 was used to support programs that had suffered federal budget cuts (Health Affairs, 2012). The use of Prevention and Public Health Fund dollars to shore up existing programs added to the controversy that had surrounded the Fund from the outset. This contributed to the $5 billion in cuts to the Fund included in the 2012 Middle Class Tax Relief and Job Creation Act. This was a major victory for Republicans, as it marked one of the first instances that the Administration and Congressional Democrats agreed to make changes—and pare back some part of the ACA.

Further fueling critics, in 2013 the Fund was used to offset costs related to exchange enrollment, as Congressionally appropriated funds were unavailable. The Department of Health and Human Services (HHS) used funds to provide enrollment support through in-person assister programs, as well as public education and outreach that included an outreach plan aimed at Hispanic Americans (Department of Health and Human Services, 2015). While the Administration made the case that supporting enrollment into exchange coverage would help prevent onset and progression of chronic diseases, supporters of the Fund were dismayed at its use. For instance, in 2013 Democratic chairman Tom Harkin (D-IA) stated:

> I was deeply disturbed, several weeks ago, to learn of the White House's plan to strip $332 million in critical funding from the Prevention and Public Health Fund and to redirect that money to educating the public about the new health insurance marketplaces and other aspects of implementing the Affordable Care Act. No one is more interested in ensuring the successful implementation of the health insurance exchanges than I am. But it is ill-advised and short-sighted to raid the Prevention Fund, which is making absolutely critical investments in preventing disease, saving lives, and

keeping women and their families healthy. . . . "I hope and expect that, going forward, the White House will respect the intent of Congress in creating the Prevention Fund in the first place, as a critical feature of the law. I expect the administration to join with us in fighting for the Prevention Fund and in making smart, evidence-based investments in prevention and wellness. This is what real health reform is about. It is our best bet for creating a healthier and more prosperous nation." (Harkin, 2013)

Efforts to defund the Prevention and Public Health Fund have continued, with bills introduced in each Congress to strip the funding altogether from the law. Representative Joe Pitts (R-PA) reintroduced such legislation in 2015:

A public health slush fund was just one of the many bad ideas contained in Obamacare. . . . Public health spending should be closely monitored by Congress. Instead, we have given the executive branch extraordinary power to spend billions of dollars without any oversight. (Pitts, 2015)

These efforts are likely to continue, although the Fund has continued to make investments in the way Congress originally envisioned, in addition to filling gaps for other issues that Congress has refused funding for. For instance, grants have been made to support tobacco cessation programs, obesity prevention efforts, state public health infrastructure and capacity, and workplace wellness grants, among other efforts (Trust for America's Health, 2013). While the Prevention and Public Health Fund has been used for many of its intended purposes, the flexibility Congress afforded it has led to its use for unintended purposes—and opening it up to charges that it has become a slush fund for the Administration.

FURTHER READING

Anderson, G. 2010. "Chronic Care: Making the Case for Ongoing Care." Robert Wood Johnson Foundation and the Johns Hopkins Bloomberg School of Public Health. Accessed March 30, 2015. http://www.rwjf.org/content/dam/farm/reports/reports/2010/rwjf54583.

Centers for Disease Control and Prevention. 2015. "Death and Mortality." NCHS FastStats. Accessed October 9, 2015. http://www.cdc.gov/nchs/fastats/deaths.htm.

Department of Health and Human Services. 2013. "The Affordable Care Act and the Prevention and Public Health Fund Report to Congress for FY2013." Accessed March 30, 2015. http://www.hhs.gov/sites/default/files/open/prevention/fy-2013-aca-pphf-report-to-congress.pdf.

Department of Health and Human Services. 2015. "Prevention and Public Health Trust Fund." Accessed March 29, 2015. http://www.hhs.gov/open/prevention/index.html.

H.R. 3630. 2012. "Middle Class Tax Relief and Job Creation Act of 2012." Accessed March 29, 2015. https://www.congress.gov/bill/112th-congress/house-bill/3630/text.

Harkin, T. 2013. "Statement by Senator Tom Harkin on the Importance of the Prevention Fund to Save Lives and Money." Senate Health Education Labor and Pensions Committee. Accessed March 30, 2015. http://www.help.senate.gov/newsroom/press/release/?id=98d8956a-8907-48f5-9547-6e98fadb618e.

Health Affairs. 2012. "The Prevention and Public Health Fund." Health Policy Briefs. Accessed March 30, 2015. http://www.healthaffairs.org/healthpolicybriefs/brief.php?brief_id=63.

Lambrew, J., and Podesta, J. 2006. "Promoting Prevention and Preempting Costs: A New Wellness Trust for the United States." Center for American Progress. Accessed March 30, 2015. https://cdn.americanprogress.org/wp-content/uploads/issues/2006/10/pdf/health_lambrew.pdf.

Office of Management and Budget. 2011. "Statement of Administration Policy: H.R. 1217—Repeal of the Affordable Care Act's Prevention and Public Health Fund." Accessed March 29, 2015. https://www.whitehouse.gov/sites/default/files/omb/legislative/sap/112/saphr1217h_20110413.pdf.

Pitts, J. 2015. "Pitts Reintroduces Bill to Eliminate Health Slush Fund." Accessed March 30, 2015. http://pitts.house.gov/press-release/pitts-reintroduces-bill-eliminate-health-slush-fund.

S. 3674. 2008. "21st Century Wellness Trust Act." Congress.gov. Accessed March 30, 2015. https://www.congress.gov/bill/110th-congress/senate-bill/3674.

Trust for America's Health. 2008. "Prevention for a Healthier America: Investments in Disease Prevention Yield Significant Savings, Stronger Communities." Accessed March 30, 2015. http://healthyamericans.org/reports/prevention08/Prevention08.pdf.

Trust for America's Health. 2013. "The Truth about the Prevention and Public Health Fund." Accessed March 30, 2015. http://healthyamericans.org/assets/files/Truth%20about%20the%20Prevention%20and%20Public%20Health%20Fund.pdf.

Q34. WILL THE UNITED STATES PREVENTIVE SERVICES TASK FORCE'S ROLE IN PREVENTION COVERAGE LEAD TO RATIONING OF HEALTH CARE?

Answer: No, it merely provides safeguards to ensure that preventive care services that were expanded under the ACA—primarily by removing cost-sharing requirements—are helpful and effective. In fact, the ACA has increased access to preventive health services for millions.

The Facts: One of the most impactful prevention-related provisions in the ACA was coverage for preventive services with no cost-sharing. But the ACA limited its coverage of preventive care services only to those services that the United States Preventive Services Task Force (USPSTF), and a few other regulatory bodies, rated as effective (i.e., an "A" or "B" rating). The ACA sought to eliminate co-pays, a primary barrier to accessing effective preventive services.

However, the USPSTF's activity proved to be controversial starting with an update to mammography screening standards in the fall of 2009. As the Senate took up debate on the ACA, the USPSTF did not recommend routine screening for women in their 40s not at risk for breast cancer. This decision spurred charges that the Task Force would engage in rationing and that the Administration's primary aim was to save costs through health reform—even though economic considerations are not to be taken into account when making recommendations about the efficacy of preventive services (American College of Radiology, 2009). In addition, there have been ongoing concerns that requiring coverage with no cost-sharing from some services would raise premiums for everyone (Gottlieb, 2011).

The ACA requires private health plans to cover effective preventive services with no cost-sharing for individuals. This provision is not only one of the most critical prevention-related measures in the law, but it has also been one of the most impactful in terms of the numbers of Americans it has applied to. The impetus behind the provision was to increase access to, and utilization of, effective preventive services, which research has shown can reduce mortality and improve health, by eliminating cost as a barrier. A research study examined both the health benefits and costs of providing 20 proven preventive services, such as tobacco cessation screening and daily aspirin use, and found that greater use of these services could save two million life-years annually and increasing use of these services to a 90 percent utilization rate would save $3.7 billion (Maciosek, 2010). By eliminating cost barriers, such as co-pays, lawmakers hoped that more people would access effective preventive services that could improve health and even save lives.

A primary point of controversy was how to determine whether a preventive service was effective in improving public health. The Maciosek study relied on those services the USPSTF recommended for the general population to define "proven" services (Maciosek, 2010). Established in 1984, the USPSTF is "an independent, volunteer panel of national experts in prevention and evidence-based medicine" whose goal is to improve health by making "evidence-based recommendations" about the use of preventive services (U.S. Preventive Services Task Force, 2014).

The ACA used a similar definition by requiring that preventive services with an A or B rating by the USPSTF (in addition to a few other groups) be covered by private insurance plans with no cost-sharing. If a service receives an A or B rating, it means that the USPSTF recommends the service. An A rating is defined as having "high certainty that the net benefit is substantial," and a B rating is defined as having "high certainty that the net benefit is moderate or there is moderate certainty that the net benefit is moderate to substantial" (U.S. Preventive Services Task Force, 2014). Critics of this ACA provision felt that the preventive services coverage requirements put new authority in the hands of the USPSTF to control the services people received.

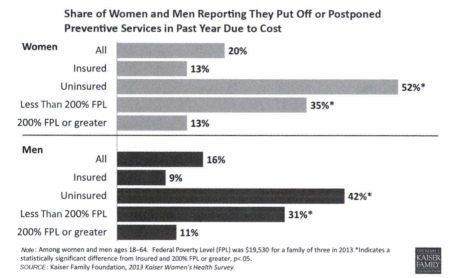

Figure 7.1 Cost Barriers to Use of Preventive Services for Women and Men

Source: Henry J. Kaiser Family Foundation. 2014. "Preventive Services Covered by Private Health Plans under the Affordable Care Act." Accessed March 31, 2015. http://kff.org/health-reform/fact-sheet/preventive-services-covered-by-private-health-plans/.

First, critics charged that this ACA requirement would allow the USPSTF to determine which services patients would receive, leading to rationing care. Second, they charged that the new coverage requirements would raise health insurance premiums in the absence of patient cost-sharing. Dr. Scott Gottlieb, a former official in the George W. Bush Administration, wrote,

> Under the Patient Protection and Affordable Care Act (PPACA), a previously obscure government advisory body has acquired vast authority to decide which health care services Americans will have access to. . . . PPACA gives the USPSTF's recommendations the force of law, making them de facto mandates on which preventive services private health plans and public programs such as Medicare must pay for. Services that do not make the USPSTF grade are unlikely to be covered at all. . . . Moreover, because the USPSTF has few guidelines governing its function, it has great flexibility to adapt its criteria and grow its mandate in ways that may conflict with political goals and public sentiment and lead to unintended consequences. (Gottlieb, 2011)

The charges of rationing in particular gained steam after the USPSTF issued a controversial recommendation on mammograms for women in their 40s not at risk for breast cancer. In 2009, as the Senate began to debate the health reform legislation, the USPSTF did not recommend routine mammograms for women in their 40s who were not at risk for breast cancer; however, it did recommend biennial mammograms for women 50 to 74 years of age. The backlash that ensued was striking—and in some cases critics alleged that the recommendation was aimed at saving costs. For instance, the American College of Radiology issued a press release, stating:

> The USPSTF recommendations are a step backward and represent a significant harm to women's health. . . . These recommendations are inconsistent with current science and apparently have been developed in an attempt to reduce costs. Unfortunately, many women may pay for this unsound approach with their lives. (American College of Radiology, 2009)

The vehemence of the attacks on the USPSTF's recommendation and its politicization "discouraged" Gail Wilensky, a well-respected Republican health policy expert, who has also championed comparative effectiveness research (Wilensky, 2010). Other experts have also weighed in about the controversy over screening recommendations and guidelines. Dating back to 2002, the USPSTF had signaled that the precise age at which mammography screening benefits outweigh risks is difficult to determine; however, when they made more nuanced recommendations related to age in 2009, it was interpreted as a "recommendation 'against' screening"— and not a discussion over weighing the relative harms and benefits for a given individual (Woolf and Harris, 2012). Unfortunately, the recommendations of a nonpartisan advisory group on which preventive services may have the greatest impact on individuals were caught in the larger claims over the ACA and how it would lead to rationing, would raise insurance premiums, and in some cases was tied to the financial impacts on these interest groups.

There is little evidence to suggest that the preventive services coverage requirements in the ACA have led to any rationing of care or worse quality or health outcomes. In fact, HHS has reported that this provision has resulted in 76 million Americans gaining coverage for expanded preventive services, and an estimated 48.5 million women benefiting from free preventive services (Burke and Simmons, 2014). Even those in employer-sponsored plans experienced an increase in benefits, with approximately two-thirds of large employers supporting the new ACA provision (AcademyHealth, 2011). Finally, while the preventive service coverage requirements did likely raise premium costs in the short run, the cost has been minimal (and may be outweighed by long-term health improvement and potential savings). In fact, one study estimated that the cost of a number of new ACA coverage requirements, including extending dependent coverage up to 26 years of age, restrictions on annual coverage limits, prohibitions on lifetime limits, and the preventive services coverage requirement altogether, may have accounted for 1 to 2 percent of overall health plan cost increases observed in 2011 (AcademyHealth, 2011).

While it is too early to assess the health and cost impacts of the preventive services coverage requirements, they have not led to rationing or a significant increase in health insurance premiums. To the contrary, evidence indicates that over 76 million Americans became newly eligible for preventive services as a result of this provision (Burke and Simmons, 2014). For most Americans with private insurance, financial barriers to preventive services have been removed (Henry J. Kaiser Family Foundation, 2014).

FURTHER READING

AcademyHealth. 2011. "The Affordable Care Act and Employer-Sponsored Insurance for Working Americans." Accessed April 1, 2015. http://www.academyhealth.org/files/nhpc/2011/AH_2011AffordableCareRe portFINAL3.pdf.

American College of Radiology. 2009. "USPSTF Mammography Recommendations Will Result in Countless Unnecessary Breast Cancer Deaths Each Year. Position Statements." Accessed March 31, 2015. http://www.acr.org/About-Us/Media-Center/Position-Statements/Position-Statements-Folder/USPSTF-Mammography-Recommen dations-Will-Result-in-Countless-Unnecessary-Breast-Cancer-Deaths.

Burke, A., and Simmons, A. 2014. "Increased Coverage of Preventive Services with Zero Cost Sharing under the Affordable Care Act." Assistant Secretary for Planning and Evaluation. Accessed March 31, 2015. http://aspe.hhs.gov/health/reports/2014/PreventiveServices/ib_ PreventiveServices.pdf.

Gottlieb, S. 2011. "The Bleeding Edge of Rationing." American Enterprise Institute. Accessed March 31, 2015. http://www.aei.org/publication/the-bleeding-edge-of-rationing/.

Henry J. Kaiser Family Foundation. 2014. "Preventive Services Covered by Private Health Plans under the Affordable Care Act." Accessed March 31, 2015. http://kff.org/health-reform/fact-sheet/preventive-ser vices-covered-by-private-health-plans/.

Maciosek, Michael V. 2010. "Greater Use of Preventive Services in U.S. Health Care Could Save Lives at Little or No Cost." *Health Affairs* 29, 9: 1656–1660.

U.S. Preventive Services Task Force. 2014. "About the USPSTF." Accessed April 1, 2015. http://www.uspreventiveservicestaskforce.org/Page/Name/about-the-uspstf.

Wilensky, G. 2010. "The Mammography Guidelines and Evidence-based Medicine." *Health Affairs Blog*. Accessed April 1, 2015. http://health affairs.org/blog/2010/01/12/the-mammograpy-guidelines-and-evidence-based-medicine/.

Woolf, S., and Harris, R. 2012. "The Harms of Screening: New Attention to an Old Concern." *Journal of the American Medical Association*, 307, 6: 565–566.

Q35. WILL THE AFFORDABLE CARE ACT WORSEN PHYSICIAN SHORTAGES AND LEAD TO LONGER WAIT TIMES FOR MEDICAL CARE?

Answer: Most studies indicate that Obamacare has not appreciably exacerbated these problems. Other factors, such as increasing health care needs of an aging American population, are cited as much bigger contributors to these issues.

The Facts: When first passed, the ACA was projected to expand coverage to 32 million Americans (Congressional Budget Office, 2010). Opponents of the law claimed that the impact of these formerly uninsured individuals gaining coverage would translate to long waiting times and shortages of physicians and providers. As evidence, critics pointed to longer wait times in Massachusetts after the state undertook health reform in 2006. Since the ACA's passage, they have continued to warn that the influx of newly insured lives, coupled with the provider payment reforms in the ACA, will put a serious strain on, and shortage of, providers (Anderson, 2014). For instance, Dr. Amy Anderson published an issue brief with the conservative Heritage Foundation writing:

> The ACA's attempts to address the shortage are unproven and limited in scope, and the significant financial investment will not produce results for years due to the training pipeline. With the ACA's estimated 190 million hours of paperwork annually imposed on businesses and the health care industry, combined with shortages of workers, patients will be facing increasing wait times, limited access to providers, shortened time with caregivers, and decreased satisfaction. The health care workforce is facing increased stress and instability, and a major redesign of the workforce is needed to extend care to millions of Americans. (Anderson, 2014)

Conservative think tanks have also cited surveys of longer wait times since the ACA's passage, but the time frame of the surveys predated the ACA's coverage expansion, calling the predictions into question (Perry, 2009).

Projections of physician shortages predate the passage of the ACA. The American Association of Medical Colleges (AAMC) has been predicting physician shortages due to general population demographic trends and physician demographic trends for years, with the most recent numbers suggesting a shortage of 45,000 to over 90,000 by 2025 (IHS, 2015). However, a recent Institute of Medicine study called the severity of these projected shortages into question (Institute of Medicine, 2014). Finally, closer examinations of wait times following health reform in Massachusetts indicate that while there was an increase in wait times generally in the initial years after health reform, unmet need had actually fallen to pre-health reform levels in the state by 2009 (Long, 2010). While physician shortages in some specialties—especially primary care—are likely due to an aging population, widespread shortages primarily due to the ACA are overstated.

In 2010, CBO projected that 32 million people would gain insurance as a result of the ACA through 2019 (Congressional Budget Office, 2010). While that number has been adjusted downward for a number of reasons, including the now voluntary nature of the Medicaid expansion, the claim that the millions of people gaining insurance would lead to long wait times and worsen physician shortages has persisted. Concerns that millions of individuals gaining coverage, many of whom had no regular source of care, would unleash "pent-up demand" and drive more people to physicians and decrease access for those with insurance were widespread. The idea that health reform would worsen the physician shortage and lead to long wait times had its origins as early as 2009, drawing on experiences in Massachusetts. The Bay State had passed major health reform in 2006, leading to the lowest uninsured rate in the nation. By the time national health reform efforts were under way, Massachusetts's experience was used by both sides as signs of success or failure on a wide range of issues. In this case, opponents used early data on wait times in the state to project national impacts. One economist examined average wait times in days for five specialties across 15 metropolitan areas, including Boston (Perry, 2009). The analysis found that Boston had the longest average weight time by 22 days compared to the next metropolitan area with the longest wait time, noting:

> Long appointment wait times in Boston also may signal what could happen nationally in the event that access to health care is expanded through health care reform. Increased demand resulting from improved access to care for approximately 47 million uninsured people can be expected to extend doctor appointment wait times in many markets. (Perry, 2009)

The charges that the ACA would have negative impacts on the provider workforce continued after the coverage expansion launched in 2014. A Heritage Foundation report predicted that the ACA would worsen existing provider shortages and "result in increased morbidity and mortality" for already underserved populations, such as rural Americans (Anderson, 2014). The charge levied was a serious one in the report—that the ACA would actually lead to more deaths due to diminished access to care, rather than improve health and reduce mortality by more people gaining insurance and access.

The concern that the ACA would worsen physician shortages was also rooted in long-standing projections by the AAMC, among other groups. AAMC commissioned reports on physician supply and demand in 2008, 2010, and again in 2015. The most recent report concluded that demand for physicians would outstrip supply between now and 2025, resulting in a shortage of 46,100 to 90,400 physicians (IHS, 2015). While the projections were still sizable, they are lower than 2010 estimates of a shortfall of 130,600 (IHS, 2015). The model used to predict physician supply and demand takes into account a number of factors, including changes in population and demographics, use of managed care, advanced practice nurses, and the ACA. When the report isolated the impact of the ACA on physician demand, it increased demand only by 2 percent over the demand increase from demographics shift alone (IHS, 2015). This suggests that broader population trends are driving health care demand and utilization in the coming years, significantly more than health reform.

A closer look at demographic trends illustrates why this is a more critical variable in physician supply and demand than the ACA. The American population will age considerably by 2050, which will be the main driver of demand for health care services and utilization. From 2015 to 2050, the percentage of the U.S. populations 65 years of age or older will increase from 15 to over 22 percent—or one in five Americans (United States Census Bureau, 2014).

Additional studies emerging from Massachusetts and following the first year of the ACA's coverage expansion also suggest that, if anything, health reform has increased access to care—and not led to unreasonable increases in wait times or adverse patient outcomes. A 2010 analysis of health reform's impacts on Massachusetts found that more adults saw physicians and fewer had unmet health needs than before health reform in the state, with especially high increases in use of preventive care and prescription

Figure 7.2 Percentage of Americans Aged 65 or Older

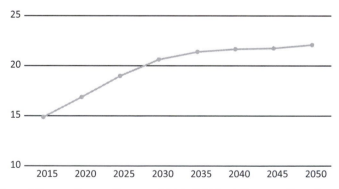

Source: United States Census Bureau, 2014. "Table 6. Percent Distribution of the Projected Population by Sex and Selected Age Groups for the United States: 2015 to 2060." Accessed April 5, 2015. http://www.census.gov/ population/projections/data/national/2014/summarytables.html.

drugs (Long, 2010). The analysis also examined impacts of health reform in the state on provider capacity. While existing wait times in Massachusetts worsened in the initial years after health reform, the trend had reversed by fall 2009 due to a number of state initiatives, including primary care physician recruitment programs, expanded medical school enrollment, and loan repayment programs for community health centers (CHCs) (Long, 2010). If Massachusetts is to be used as an example for what could happen nationally, initial exacerbations in wait times could be abated within a few years with the appropriate initiatives in place to strengthen primary care and loan repayment programs, many of which the ACA includes.

To assess the effects of the ACA on provider practices, the Robert Wood Johnson Foundation and athena Research have launched a new research initiative—ACAView. A recent report assessing whether primary care physicians are seeing more new patient assessments after the ACA coverage expansion went into effect shows mixed results. There was some indication in the later part of 2014 that physicians were establishing new patient relationships at higher rates than before 2014; however, there were no indications of excessively long wait times or physician shortages (athenaResearch, 2014).

Interestingly, the profile of new patients seen also suggests similar clinical intensity and levels of chronic disease, suggesting that those who gained insurance and accessed physicians in 2014 did not have greater health needs than those already in the system (athenaResearch, 2014).

To summarize, the claims that the ACA will lead to longer wait times and worsen physician shortages had some legitimate origins; however, it was also used to make people with insurance fearful of diminished access as millions of the uninsured gained coverage. The likely driver of any physician shortages or wait times in the future is largely due to an aging population—and not the uninsured gaining coverage through the ACA.

FURTHER READING

Anderson, A. 2014. "The Impact of the Affordable Care Act on the Health Care Workforce." The Heritage Foundation. Accessed April 2, 2015. http://www.heritage.org/research/reports/2014/03/the-impact-of-the-affordable-care-act-on-the-health-care-workforce.

athenaResearch. 2014. "ACAView: Tracking the Impact of Affordable Care." Robert Wood Johnson Foundation, Athenahealth. Accessed April 5, 2015. http://www.athenahealth.com/_doc/pdf/ACAView_Final_Comprehensive_Report.pdf.

Congressional Budget Office. 2010. "Letter to the Honorable Nancy Pelosi on H.R. 4872, the Reconciliation Act of 2010." March 20, 2010.

Accessed April 2, 2015. https://www.cbo.gov/sites/default/files/cbofiles/ftpdocs/113xx/doc11379/amendreconprop.pdf.

IHS. 2015. "The Complexities of Physician Supply and Demand: Projections from 2013 to 2025." Accessed April 2, 2015. https://www.aamc.org/download/426242/data/ihsreportdownload.pdf.

Institute of Medicine. 2014. *Graduate Medical Education that Meets the Nation's Needs.* National Academies Press: Washington, DC. http://www.nap.edu/openbook.php?record_id=18754&page=R1.

Long, S. 2010. "What Is the Evidence on Health Reform in Massachusetts and How Might the Lessons from Massachusetts Apply to National Health Reform?" The Urban Institute. Accessed April 2, 2015. http://www.urban.org/uploadedpdf/412118-massachusetts-national-health-reform.pdf.

Perry, M. 2009. "Obamacare = Longer Wait Times; Exhibit A: MASS." American Enterprise Institute. Accessed April 5, 2015. https://www.aei.org/publication/obamacare-longer-wait-times-exhibit-a-mass/.

United States Census Bureau, 2014. "Table 6. Percent Distribution of the Projected Population by Sex and Selected Age Groups for the United States: 2015 to 2060." Accessed April 5, 2015. http://www.census.gov/population/projections/data/national/2014/summarytables.html.

Q36. DOES THE AFFORDABLE CARE ACT FORCE EMPLOYERS TO PROVIDE CONTRACEPTION COVERAGE AND FUND ABORTIONS?

Answer: Contraception and abortion are two of the most controversial issues in health care—and the ACA was not immune to the debate over access to either from the start. The firestorm over access to contraception led to a Supreme Court case, widely known as the *Hobby Lobby* case, over whether closely held corporations had to make contraception available to employees at no cost to comply with the preventive services coverage requirement. In that case, a bitterly divided Supreme Court ruled that the ownership of such companies could choose not to offer contraception coverage if doing so violated their religious beliefs.

Similarly, abortion also became a hot button issue in the ACA with charges that the law funds abortions. To try to avoid an abortion-related debate during health reform, lawmakers applied the long-standing Hyde Amendment, which prohibits the use of federal funds for abortion unless the pregnancy is a result of rape or incest, or the woman's life is in danger. In addition, the ACA does not preempt state abortion laws, such as waiting periods or parental consent or notification (Salganicoff, Beames-derfer, and Kurani, 2014). However, the claims that the ACA would fund abortions—and increase funding to abortion providers—have continued.

The Facts: When crafting the legislation that eventually became the Affordable Care Act, Democratic lawmakers and officials in the Obama Administration intended contraception coverage to be one of the effective preventive services that was to be made available to individuals with no cost-sharing in both individual and group (or employer) health plans. While this provision aimed to increase access to preventive services by guaranteeing coverage and removing financial barriers to accessing effective services, contraception coverage in particular became very controversial.

Conservatives rallied against the contraception requirement—*The Daily Signal*, a Heritage Foundation blog, claimed it violated religious freedom:

> These Americans rightly argue that Obamacare is threatening their ability to work and serve in accordance with their values by forcing them to provide coverage of life-ending drugs and devices in violation of their moral or religious beliefs. (Torre, 2013)

On the other hand, supporters of the law and contraception rights felt that the ACA guaranteed access and reduced barriers to obtaining contraception for all women—regardless of payer.

Soon after the law's passage, the HHS issued regulations on coverage for effective preventive services, including FDA-approved methods with no cost-sharing, but not for drugs to induce abortions or services related to male reproduction (Healthcare.gov, 2015). The regulations affected group health plans, which touched off a firestorm among religiously affiliated employers. In response, HHS amended the original regulations exempting group health plans that were established or maintained by religious employers, and later issued "accommodations" for religiously affiliated nonprofit organizations, which could include religiously affiliated universities and health care providers. However, private companies—or those "closely held," meaning that they were not publicly traded companies—were not exempt from the requirement, triggering a number of lawsuits. The most high-profile case, *Hobby Lobby v. Burwell*, was taken up by the Supreme Court in March 2014. The Court ruled in favor of *Hobby Lobby*, maintaining that closely held private companies could choose not to offer contraception coverage if doing so violated their religious beliefs. When the provision is examined from legislation to implementation, employers are not forced to offer contraception services to their employees as a result of HHS's regulations for religiously affiliated employers and the Supreme Court decision.

The abortion provisions in the ACA and enduring problems following implementation are more complicated than even the contraception issue. The ACA included a number of provisions aimed at preventing an abortion debate over health reform—and to allow pro-life Democrats to vote for the law, which was necessary to ensure passage. First, the ACA reinforces the Hyde Amendment, which has prohibited the use of federal funds for abortion (unless the pregnancy is the result of rape or incest, or the woman's life is in danger) since 1977. Second, the law does not preempt any state abortions laws, such as parental consent or notification or waiting periods. Third, the ACA allows states to prohibit coverage for any abortion services in their exchanges, which 25 states have done (Salganicoff, Beamesderfer, and Kurani, 2014). Finally, to ensure that federal funds are not used for abortion, the ACA also required that there be segregation of funds so that only private funds could be used to pay for the cost of abortion coverage.

Segregation of funds was a complicated solution arrived at in the Senate to maintain access to abortion services in the health exchanges, but only through patient premium contributions (and not federal subsidies). The ACA requires that any plan that covers abortion services must pay at least $1 per month into a segregated fund that would be used to pay for abortion services. To address the concerns of those who would not want any of their premium dollars to go to a segregated fund, the ACA requires that exchanges in all states offer a coverage option that does not include any abortion services. Unfortunately, the compromise did not satisfy either side. Abortion rights groups opposed the language, although not the ACA itself, because it would lead to "unacceptable bureaucratic stigmatization (that) could cause insurance carriers to drop abortion coverage, even though more than 85 percent of private plans currently cover this care for women" (NARAL, 2010). Pro-life groups expressed opposition not only to the segregation of funds solution but to the law itself. The United States Conference of Catholic Bishops urged members of the House of Representatives to vote against the Senate legislation (United States Conference of Catholic Bishops, 2010). While neither side was satisfied with the arrangement, abortion rights groups felt the gains from insuring millions of the uninsured outweighed restrictions or diminished access to abortion in private plans.

Given these complexities, all of these solutions were fraught with controversy throughout the debate, with pro-life Democrats struggling to support the law up until its passage. Perhaps the most notable situation arose with Rep. Bart Stupak (D-MI), who represented a key voting bloc of pro-life Democrats who were necessary to pass the Senate's ACA through the House in March 2010. The group felt that the Senate legislation did not effectively prohibit the use of federal funds for abortion services. In response, on the day of the ACA's passage in the House, President Obama announced he would issue an Executive Order reinforcing that the Hyde Amendment would apply to coverage in the health insurance exchanges (The White House, 2010). While pro-choice groups did not support the Executive Order, at least one supported the ACA overall because it would extend coverage to millions of uninsured Americans:

> For more than a year, Planned Parenthood has worked tirelessly for a health care reform bill that would fix our broken health care system, strengthen women's health, and achieve quality, affordable health care for all Americans. Today, monumental progress was made toward achieving these goals with the passage of historic health care reform legislation by the U.S. House of Representatives, despite a symbolic gesture, in the form of an Executive Order, to anti-choice Congressman Bart Stupak (D-MI), which has diverted attention from the central goal of health care reform—controlling costs and extending coverage. (Planned Parenthood, 2010)

Obama's executive order satisfied Stupak, who eventually voted in favor of the ACA (and may have lost his bid for reelection in November 2010 as a result of that vote). Indeed, the controversy over abortion, much like the controversy over contraception, did not disappear after the law's passage. Allegations that the ACA supported abortion services continued. For instance, when HHS announced that recipients for Navigator and in-person assister grants included Planned Parenthood, conservative critics assailed the decision, contending that it would increase funding to an abortion provider despite the protections in the law (Torre, 2013).

One analysis estimated that over one-third of women who became eligible for coverage because of the ACA's coverage expansion could enroll only in plans that were subject to the Hyde Amendment or more restrictive policies (Salganicoff, Beamesderfer, and Kurani, 2014). The additional requirements for providing or offering abortion services may also act as a deterrent for payers moving forward. At this time, the ACA does not appear to expand access to abortion through the use of federal funds to subsidize abortion coverage or by increasing access by preempting state law.

FURTHER READING

Healthcare.gov. 2015. "Birth Control Benefits." Accessed May 26, 2015. https://www.healthcare.gov/coverage/birth-control-benefits.

NARAL. 2010. "Statement on Health Reform." NARAL Pro-Choice America. Accessed April 7, 2015. http://www.prochoiceamerica.org/media/press-releases/2010/pr03212010-finalhousehcr.html.

Planned Parenthood. 2010. "National News." Accessed April 7, 2015. http://www.plannedparenthood.org/about-us/newsroom/press-releases/statement-cecile-richards-president-ppfa-house-passing-historic-health-care-reform-bill.

Salganicoff, A., Beamesderfer, A., Kurani, N., and Sobel, L. 2014. "Coverage for Abortion Services and the ACA." Henry J. Kaiser Family Foundation. Accessed April 6, 2015. http://kff.org/womens-health-policy/issue-brief/coverage-for-abortion-services-and-the-aca/.

Torre, S. 2013. "Obamacare Is Restricting Choice and Trampling Religious Freedoms." *The Daily Signal.* Accessed April 6, 2015. http://dailysignal.com/2013/11/29/obamacare-restricting-choice-trampling-fundamental-freedoms/.

United States Conference of Catholic Bishops. 2010. "Letter to House of Representatives on Health Reform Bill." Accessed April 7, 2015. http://www.usccb.org/issues-and-action/human-life-and-dignity/health-care/letter-to-house-of-representatives-from-dinardo-murphy-wester-on-health-reform-bill-2010-03-20.cfm.

The White House. 2010. "Executive Order 13535—Patient Protection and Affordable Care Act's Consistency with Longstanding Restrictions on the Use of Federal Funds for Abortion." Accessed April 7, 2015. https://www.whitehouse.gov/the-press-office/executive-order-patient-protection-and-affordable-care-acts-consistency-with-longst.

Q37. WILL THE AFFORDABLE CARE ACT IMPROVE THE OVERALL HEALTH OF THE AMERICAN PEOPLE?

Answer: Unknown at this point. Supporters, however, are confident that as the number of people without health insurance—and thus, as a practical matter, without access to health care—continues to decline under the ACA, and as the ACA's preventive services provisions become more entrenched, meaningful improvements in various health measurements will become apparent.

The Facts: The end goal of reducing the ranks of the uninsured is to increase access to health care services that will improve population health. For years, the U.S. health system has ranked behind other industrialized nations on numerous factors, including life expectancy (Commonwealth Fund, 2014; Murray and Frenk, 2010; OECD, 2014). Yet America's per capita health care costs were the highest in the world at $8,915 in 2012 (Centers for Medicare and Medicaid Services, 2014). This state of affairs existed to a significant degree because in 2010, when the ACA passed, 50 million Americans were uninsured (Centers for Medicare and Medicaid Services, 2014; DeNavas, Proctor, and Smith, 2010; OECD, 2014). Lower-income Americans tended to have higher rates of uninsurance, shorter life expectancies, higher rates of obesity, and fewer preventive procedures, such as colorectal screenings than higher-income counterparts (Department of Health and Human Services, 2011). These sharply striking statistics underscore one of the primary drivers for health reform—to improve health outcomes and status by expanding access to insurance.

Opponents of the ACA alleged that the opposite would be true—that the law would actually lead to higher rates of mortality and other negative health consequences because it would reduce access to providers (Anderson, 2014). In particular, conservative critics of the law focus on Medicaid, claiming that expansion will actually worsen health outcomes due to restricted access in the program in many parts of the country. The American Legislative Exchange Council (ALEC), a right-leaning membership organization of state legislators, charged:

> The Patient Protection and Affordable Care Act will mire states in a poorly designed Medicaid program and will lead to skyrocketing enrollment in government-run health care and untenable state budgets. Their citizens, meanwhile, will face restricted access to care and worsening health outcomes. (American Legislative Exchange Council, 2011)

President Obama and his Democratic supporters in Congress rejected these forecasts, and they framed the ACA as a vehicle for getting American health care on a better course. But even advocates of the ACA acknowledged that the challenge is considerable.

The Commonwealth Fund has released several comparative analyses of the U.S. health system performance relative to that of other industrialized nations. Each updated report makes a consistent finding—that the U.S.

health care system "underperforms relative to other countries on most dimensions of performance" (Commonwealth Fund, 2014). The analysis goes on to find:

> The U.S. also ranks behind most countries on many measures of health outcomes, quality, and efficiency. U.S. physicians face particular difficulties receiving timely information, coordinating care, and dealing with administrative hassles. The U.S. ranks last overall with poor scores on all three indicators of healthy lives—mortality amenable to medical care, infant mortality, and healthy life expectancy at age 60. The U.S. and U.K. had much higher death rates in 2007 from conditions amenable to medical care than some of the other countries, e.g., rates 25 percent to 50 percent higher than Australia and Sweden. Overall, France, Sweden, and Switzerland rank highest on healthy lives. (Commonwealth Fund, 2014)

Other reports have come to the same conclusion, including the Organisation for Economic Co-operation and Development (OECD), which found that U.S. life expectancy was 1.5 years lower than the OECD average (OECD, 2014). The difference was attributed to gaps in health insurance coverage, lack of access to primary care, and poor health behaviors and living conditions (OECD, 2014). The Centers for Disease Control and Prevention have also examined the relationship between socioeconomic status and health. They found that life expectancy among the U.S. population was 9.3 years lower for men and 8.6 years lower for women without a high school diploma compared to those with bachelor's degrees or higher education (Department of Health and Human Services, 2011). The report also detailed a number of income-related disparities including higher rates of depression, obesity, and tobacco use, and lower rates of colorectal tests—and that those at lower levels of poverty more likely to be uninsured and forego medical care due to costs (Department of Health and Human Services, 2011). Overall, health status and outcomes do not match the amount of money the United States spends on health care.

While the ACA sought to correct this imbalance, there were critics alleging that the opposite would actually happen—that the law would worsen health status outcomes. One contributor to The Heritage Foundation alleged that the law would worsen provider shortages, especially in rural areas, and "the danger is that these shortages will result in increased morbidity and mortality for rural Americans" (Anderson, 2014). ALEC released *The State Legislators Guide to Repealing Obamacare* in 2011, which focused on a number of issues, including reasons to oppose Medicaid expansion (American Legislative Exchange Council, 2011). The group alleged that Medicaid programs were already "overburdened"—and that enrolling more individuals in the program would lead to poorer access to care and poorer health outcomes (American Legislative Exchange Council, 2011). However, the evidence to date does not support the claim that the ACA has restricted access or overburdened providers to the point that it has caused patient harm.

In fact, early research studies are showing improvement in the health care delivery system and preliminary improvement in health status in some cases. First, the payment and delivery reforms in the law are changing the health care delivery system, resulting in an estimated 150,000 fewer preventable readmissions into hospitals for Medicare beneficiaries and fewer hospital-acquired conditions resulting in 50,000 prevented deaths and $12 billion in savings (Blumenthal, Abrams, and Nuzum, 2015). In terms of health status changes, one study comparing health trends in Massachusetts, where health reform was passed in 2006, with neighboring states from 2001 to 2011 found that Massachusetts' residents reported greater improvements in physical and mental health, and had significantly higher rates of preventive services such as colonoscopies and cholesterol testing (Van Der Wees, Zaslavksy, and Ayanian, 2013). Another study examined the impacts of expanding Medicaid on medical outcomes and found that there were some improved outcomes with more low-income individuals gaining coverage, such as diagnosis of diabetes and use of diabetes medication, and improved use of preventive services (Baicker et al., 2013).

These and other studies provide little evidence to suggest that the ACA has worsened health outcomes; in fact, early research is suggesting that providing insurance coverage leads to more people seeking preventive services and improvements in health outcomes (Baicker et al., 2013). The long-term impact of the ACA on health status and outcomes will take years to evaluate, but early evidence indicates that positive impacts on health are being observed.

FURTHER READING

American Legislative Exchange Council. 2011. "The State Legislators Guide to Repealing ObamaCare." Accessed April 8, 2015. http://www .alec.org/wp-content/uploads/State_Leg_Guide_to_Repealing_Obama Care.pdf.

Anderson, A. 2014. "The Impact of the Affordable Care Act on the Health Care Workforce." The Heritage Foundation. Accessed April 2, 2015. http://www.heritage.org/research/reports/2014/03/the-impact-of-the-affordable-care-act-on-the-health-care-workforce.

Baicker, K., Taubman, S., Allen, H., Bernstein, M., Gruber, J., Newhouse, J., Schneider, E., Wright, B., Zaslavsky, A., and Finkelstein, A. 2013. "The Oregon Experiment—Effects of Medicaid on Clinical Outcomes." *The New England Journal of Medicine*, 368: 1713–1722.

Blumenthal, D., Abrams, M., and Nuzum, R. 2015. "The Affordable Care Act at 5 Years." *The New England Journal of Medicine, Health Policy Report*. Accessed May 28, 2015. http://www.nejm.org/doi/full/10.1056/NEJMhpr1503614.

Centers for Medicare and Medicaid Services. 2014. "National Health Expenditure Projections 2012–2022." Accessed April 8, 2014. http://www.cms.gov/Research-Statistics-Data-and-Systems/Statistics-Trends-and-Reports/NationalHealthExpendData/Downloads/tables.pdf.

Commonwealth Fund. 2014. "Mirror, Mirror on the Wall, 2014 Update: How the U.S. Health Care System Compares Internationally." Accessed April 9, 2015. http://www.commonwealthfund.org/publications/fund-reports/2014/jun/mirror-mirror.

Department of Health and Human Services. 2011. "Health, United States, 2011." Centers for Disease Control and Prevention. National Center for Health Statistics. Accessed May 26, 2015. http://www.cdc.gov/nchs/data/hus/hus11.pdf.

DeNavas, C., Proctor, B., and Smith, J. 2011. "Income, Poverty, and Health Insurance Coverage in the United States: 2010." United States Census Bureau. Accessed February 28, 2015. http://www.census.gov/prod/2011pubs/p60-239.pdf.

Murray, C., and Frenk, J. 2010. "Ranking 37th—Measuring the Performance of the U.S. Health Care System." *New England Journal of Medicine*, 362: 98–99.

OECD. 2014. "OECD Health Statistics 2014: How Does the United States Compare?" Accessed April 8, 2015. http://www.oecd.org/unitedstates/Briefing-Note-UNITED-STATES-2014.pdf.

Van Der Wees, P., Zaslavksy, A., and Ayanian, J. 2013. "Improvements in Health Status after Massachusetts Health Care Reform." *Milbank Quarterly*, 91, 4: 663–689. Accessed May 26, 2015. http://www.milbank.org/uploads/documents/featured-articles/pdf/Volume91_Issue4_Improvements_in_Health_Status_after_Massachusetts_Health_Care_Reform.pdf.

Q38. WILL THE AFFORDABLE CARE ACT STRENGTHEN PRIMARY CARE?

Answer: Primary care is often the first point of entry into the medical system. A strong primary care system is necessary for the overall health system to be both effective and efficient (Health Resources and Services Administration, 2013). However, primary care in the United States has been weakening over the past several decades for political, scientific, and economic reasons (Sandy et al., 2009). Unfortunately, this decline is a major contributor to the cost and quality problems plaguing the health system. One of the many ways the ACA tried to improve quality and reduce costs was to strengthen primary care through a number of mechanisms in the law, including encouraging the implementation of patient-centered medical homes (PCMHs), temporarily increasing Medicaid payments to primary care providers, workforce training and loan repayment programs aimed at increasing the number of primary care providers, and additional funding for Federally Qualified Health Centers. While it is too early to tell how the ACA will impact primary care in America over the long term, early evidence suggests that primary care has been strengthened, with payers and health systems focusing on the foundational role it plays in care delivery.

The Facts: Primary care consists of general and family medicine, pediatrics, internal medicine, and geriatrics, and can include physicians as well as nurse practitioners and physician assistants trained in primary care specialties (Health Resources and Services Administration, 2013). These providers are often the first points of contact in the health system and serve the broadest patient population, but less than one-third of all physicians in the United States specialize in primary care (Agency for Health Care Research and Quality, 2014).

The supply of primary care doctors has been on the decline in the United States for several decades—and the ensuing imbalance between primary and specialty care in the United States has been a major contributor to poor health system performance and poor health outcomes relative to other industrialized nations (Sandy et al., 2009). Reasons cited for the decline in primary care are economic, scientific, and political, including the rise of the biomedical model in medicine in the United States; the use of "relative value units" to determine physician payment, which tend to value specialty services and procedures over primary care services; and the lack of federal policy on how funding for physician training should be distributed to support an appropriate percentage of primary care physicians (Sandy et al., 2009). This steady decline in primary care capacity, which should be serving as the foundation of the health care system, has had severe consequences.

While primary care has become less central to U.S. health care delivery system, costs have skyrocketed, with the United States spending $8,915 per capita on health care in 2012—more than any other nation (Centers for Medicare and Medicaid Services, 2014). At the same time, the quality of care in the United States is not commensurate with levels of spending. A landmark study in 2003 found that Americans only receive recommended care approximately 55 percent of the time from providers (McGlynn et al., 2003), and subsequent studies have shown continued shortfalls in access to needed health care services.

In the face of these challenges, lawmakers sought to strength primary care as the foundation of the health care system in the ACA. Some of the provisions for accomplishing this include:

- an increase in Medicare and Medicaid payments for primary care services;
- new multi-payer pilots to establish PCMHs, a model in which patient care is coordinated through primary care in a way that is comprehensive, patient-centered, coordinated, accessible, and of high quality;
- loan repayment and training programs for primary care providers;
- $11 billion in funding CHCs, which are often the major primary care provider for safety net populations;
- coverage for effective preventive services with no cost-sharing.

The ACA included a broad range of measures aimed at promoting the role of primary care in coordinating patient care through new payment and care delivery models, as well as financial incentives and resources.

Meanwhile, critics contended that the ACA's goal of adding millions of previously uninsured Americans to the health care system would actually weaken primary care in the United States. The Heritage Foundation, a right-leaning think tank, alleged that the ACA would harm physicians, including primary care doctors, citing new regulations, oversight, and uncertain or inadequate reimbursements through Medicare and Medicaid (Senger, 2013). Another conservative think tank, the Cato Institute, predicted that primary care options would diminish because of the influx of new patients created by the ACA (Hentoff, 2013):

[The] health care expense problem and the vanishing of primary care doctors do not, of course, affect President Barack Obama personally.

He and his family are very well protected on health matters by our taxpayer funds. But he sure has limited the availability of health care—and actual survival prospects for many of us—while changing the future professional careers of a growing number of doctors. (Hentoff, 2013)

The Heritage Foundation cited low payment rates in Medicare and Medicaid, new quality-based payment programs, and entities such as the Patient-Centered Outcomes Research Institute and the Independent Payment Advisory Board as reasons that physicians, including primary care physicians, would be adversely impacted by the law (Senger, 2013). However, these forecasts did not provide qualitative or quantitative research or evidence to support their conclusions.

Early evidence suggests that these prognostications were erroneous, and that the ACA has actually served to strengthen primary care and its role in the health care system. The Center for Medicare and Medicaid Innovation has several primary care–focused demonstrations and programs under way, with over 1,000 primary care practices participating across the country (Center for Medicare and Medicaid Innovation, 2015). The Administration has provided funding to train approximately 2,300 new primary care providers, including residents, nurse practitioners, and physician assistants, by 2015 (The White House, 2012). Finally, while shortages that predate passage of Obamacare still abound (and are projected into the future), interest in primary care as a specialty has been on the rise since the ACA passed.

The American Academy of Family Physicians reported six straight years of increases in the number of family medicine residency positions offered and filled, and increases in internal medicine and pediatrics were also observed in 2015 (American Academy of Family Physicians, 2015; National Resident Matching Program, 2015). Payers and health systems are also showing interest in primary care, as new value-based payment models, such as accountable care organizations, require strong primary care practices to manage chronic disease and execute on population health. In fact, payers and health systems are purchasing primary care practices in an effort to drive care coordination—which is the key to succeeding under value-based payments in which providers must control costs and improve quality.

It is too early to tell if the ACA will be able to reverse, or at least stem the further decline of primary care after decades of erosion; however, early evidence suggests that the law may have sparked increased innovation in primary care, greater interest from young physicians in the specialty, and a focus on the part of payers and health systems in aligning with primary care practices because they are so critical to improving health care costs and quality.

FURTHER READING

Agency for Health care Research and Quality. 2014. "The Number of Practicing Primary Care Physicians in the United States." Accessed April 10, 2015. http://www.ahrq.gov/research/findings/factsheets/primary/pcwork1/index.html.

American Academy of Family Physicians. 2015. "2015 Match Results for Primary Care and Specialty Care." Accessed April 11, 2015. http://www.aafp.org/medical-school-residency/program-directors/nrmp/other-specialities.html.

Centers for Medicare and Medicaid Services. 2014. "National Health Expenditure Projections 2012–2022." Accessed April 8, 2014. http://www.cms.gov/Research-Statistics-Data-and-Systems/Statistics-Trends-and-Reports/NationalHealthExpendData/Downloads/tables.pdf.

Centers for Medicare and Medicaid Services. 2015. "Innovation Models." Accessed October 9, 2015. http://innovation.cms.gov/initiatives/index.html#views=models&key=primary care.

Health Resources and Services Administration. 2013. "Projecting the Supply and Demand for Primary Care Practitioners through 2020." Bureau of Health Professions, National Center for Health Workforce Analysis. Accessed April 10, 2015. http://bhpr.hrsa.gov/healthworkforce/supplydemand/usworkforce/primarycare/projectingprimarycare.pdf.

Hentoff, N. 2013. "What Obamacare Can Do to You—Not for You." Cato Institute. Accessed April 10, 2015. http://www.cato.org/publications/commentary/what-obamacare-can-do-you-not-you.

McGlynn, E., Asch, S., Adams, J., Keesey, J., Hicks, J., DeCristafano, A. and Kerr, E., 2003. "The Quality of Health Care Delivered to Adults in the United States." *New England Journal of Medicine*, 348: 2635–2645. Accessed April 11, 2015. http://www.nejm.org/doi/full/10.1056/NEJMsa022615.

National Resident Matching Program. 2015. "Press Release: 2015 Residency Match Largest on Record with More Than 41,000 Applicants Vying for over 30,000 Residency Position in 4,756 Programs." Accessed April 11, 2015. http://www.nrmp.org/press-release-2015-residency-match-largest-on-record-with-more-than-41000-applicants-vying-for-over-30000-residency-positions-in-4756-programs/.

Sandy, L., Bodenheimer, T., Pawlson, G., and Starfield, B. 2009. "The Political Economy of U.S. Primary Care." *Health Affairs*, 28, 4: 1136–1145. Accessed April 11, 2015. http://content.healthaffairs.org/content/28/4/1136.full.

Senger, A. 2013. "Obamacare's Impact on Doctors—An Update." The Heritage Foundation. Accessed April 10, 2015. http://www.heritage.org/research/reports/2013/08/obamacares-impact-on-doctors-an-update.

The White House. 2012. "Creating Health Care Jobs by Addressing Primary Care Workforce Needs." Accessed April 11, 2015. https://www.whitehouse.gov/the-press-office/2012/04/11/fact-sheet-creating-health-care-jobs-addressing-primary-care-workforce-n.

8

Taxes and the Affordable Care Act

Tax policy is nearly always a politically divisive topic—and the Afford-able Care Act (ACA) brought tax policy and health reform together in particularly combustible form. The intersection of these two controversial topics created a number of opportunities for Republicans to insist that the ACA increased taxes on individuals, businesses, and employers in ways that would devastate individual families and the overall economy. The House Ways and Means Committee Republican Majority issued a press release on the taxes in the ACA, stating: "New estimates by the Congres-sional Budget Office (CBO) and the Joint Committee on Taxation (JCT) confirm what America already knows—that the Democrats' health law is a trillion-dollar tax hike that families and employers simply cannot afford" (Committee on Ways and Means, 2012). Claims that the ACA increases taxes are accurate—the ACA does increase taxes on individu-als and businesses through a number of mechanisms—but the economic impacts of the tax increases on individuals and businesses were exagger-ated in some cases.

However, the taxes in the law were included to ensure that health reform would not add to the national deficit, and also to incentivize behavior change among individuals. First, the tax revenues throughout the law help mitigate the cost of the coverage expansion through the health insurance exchanges and Medicaid expansion. Second, the indi-vidual mandate requires individuals to purchase coverage (with some exceptions) or face a penalty. The primary goal is not to raise revenues from the penalties, but to convince as many people as are able to purchase coverage. Another tax provision examined in this section is the excise tax on high-cost or "Cadillac" insurance plans, which aims to reduce the generosity of employer-sponsored insurance, which ends up raising more revenue from increased taxable income for individuals than from the excise tax itself. Republicans have targeted these tax increases and policies to voice their ongoing opposition to the ACA. And generally, it is true that the law increases taxes on individuals (especially high-income individuals) and businesses in the health care sector in particular. Defenders of the law, however, argue that this revenue is critical to ensuring that the ACA does not increase federal deficits by allowing the uninsured to purchase coverage that many found cost prohibitive previously.

Q39. DOES THE AFFORDABLE CARE ACT INCREASE TAXES ON INDIVIDUALS AND BUSINESSES?

Answer: Yes, the ACA included a number of taxes and fees—mainly on the health care industry, but also on some individuals—to help offset the cost of the ACA's coverage expansion—and even reduce the deficit. In total, the law includes approximately 15 changes in tax policies, including new taxes and fees affecting insurance companies, pharmaceutical manufacturers, medical device manufacturers, and individuals, especially high-income earners. When the law passed in 2010, the Joint Committee on Taxation (JCT) estimated that these provisions would raise $437.8 billion from 2010 to 2019 (Joint Committee on Taxation, 2010). Tax increases, however, are always controversial—and the ones included in the ACA have been no exception.

Conservative groups, such as Americans for Tax Reform, released lists of tax increases under the Obama Administration, including those in the ACA (Americans for Tax Reform, 2012). Republicans in Congress and conservative think tanks also released information on the new taxes and penalties in the law—in one case projecting the total costs of these provisions to be $836 billion to $1 trillion (Committee on Ways and Means, 2012; The Heritage Foundation, 2012). However, the amount of tax revenue the bill generates varies depending on the 10-year budget window examined—and increases over time as all the ACA's provisions go into effect and to account for inflation. The ACA does increase taxes on industry and individuals, and imposes new tax-based penalties on individuals and businesses; however, the economic impacts on businesses and individuals have been exaggerated in some cases.

The Facts: The Congressional architects of health reform were nearly all in agreement that any law they crafted had to be budget neutral—or even deficit reducing—in order for it to secure the necessary political support for passage. In other words, their health reform efforts could not add to the federal deficit—an especially critical point in 2009–2010 during the Great Recession.

In the Senate, the commitment to a budget neutral or deficit-reducing health reform bill began with the 2009 Budget Resolution, which allowed for health reform efforts that would "[be] deficit-neutral, reduce excess cost growth in health care spending and are fiscally sustainable over the long term" (S.Con.Res.13, 2009). The coverage expansion was the centerpiece of the law and of course carried the highest price tag. To cover the costs of the premium subsidies and the Medicaid expansion, the ACA included (1) Medicare provider payment reductions, (2) penalties against employers with more than 50 full-time employees that do not provide affordable coverage and against individuals who forego (but can afford) coverage, and (3) new taxes on industry and individuals—primarily high-income earners, which raised the most revenue of the three categories.

The Senate Finance Committee took the approach that the health care industry should help finance the coverage expansion in light of the benefits they would realize from more individuals having insurance and access to provider services, pharmaceutical products, and medical devices. In the end, the ACA included the following tax provisions affecting health care industry sectors:

- Health insurance companies: Insurers were subject to an annual fee starting at $6.1 billion in the first year of the coverage expansion in 2014, growing to $12.1 billion in 2019 and indexed to medical cost growth in subsequent years. From 2010 through 2019 the insurer fee raised $60.1 billion (Joint Committee on Taxation, 2010).
- Pharmaceutical manufacturers: Manufacturers and importers of brand pharmaceutical products were subject to an annual fee totaling $27 billion from 2010 through 2019 (Joint Committee on Taxation, 2010).
- Device manufacturers: Device companies were subject to a 2.3 percent excise tax on certain medical devices, totaling $20 billion in tax revenue from 2010 through 2019 (Joint Committee on Taxation, 2010).
- Indoor tanning: Indoor tanning services were subject to a 10 percent excise tax, raising $2.7 billion from 2010 through 2019 (Joint Committee on Taxation, 2010).

In total, these major industry tax provisions totaled $166.5 billion in revenue from 2013 through 2022.

Opponents of the law maintained that the industry taxes would simply be passed onto individuals—in the form of higher premiums, drug prices, or higher prices hospitals and providers would pay for devices. The right-leaning American Action Forum released an analysis that estimated that the costs of the insurer fee, pharmaceutical fee, and medical device tax together would add $130 in 2014 to the premiums of insurance purchased in the exchange, and $29 for self-insured employer plans (Book, 2014). The conservative Heritage Foundation also examined the insurer tax and concluded that the tax targeting insurers was structured in a way that the cost could easily be passed on to individual purchasers (Burton, 2013). Economists make the distinction between the entity or individual subject to the tax (known as the statutory incidence of the tax), and who actually bears the cost, or the economic incidence (Hemmings, Fangmeier, and Udow-Phillips, 2013). Economic theory suggests that the impacts of these fees are likely to be felt by consumers.

The ACA also included tax provisions aimed at individuals—especially high-income earners—to offset the cost of the coverage expansion. Some of the significant individual tax provision included:

- Medicare Hospital Insurance Tax: Increase in the Medicare Hospital Insurance (HI) tax of 0.9 percent for high-income earners (defined as individuals with earned income over $200,000 and families over $250,000; Joint Committee on Taxation, 2010).
- Unearned income: A 3.8 percent contribution on unearned income to the Medicare HI on tax high-income earners (defined as individuals with earned income over $200,000 and families over $250,000; Joint Committee on Taxation, 2010).
- Flexible Spending Accounts. Limitations on Flexible Spending Accounts (FSAs) to $2,500, indexed to grow with the Consumer Price Index (Joint Committee on Taxation, 2010).
- Medical Expenses Deduction: Increased the threshold for the medical expenses deduction from 7.5 percent of Adjusted Gross Income to 10 percent, but maintained threshold at 7.5 percent for taxpayers (or their spouses) who turn 65 years of age from 2013 through 2016 (Joint Committee on Taxation, 2010).

In total, these provisions raised $360.4 billion in revenue from 2013 through 2022, with nearly 90 percent of the revenue coming from the

HI taxes for high-income earners (Congressional Budget Office, 2012). Finally, another controversial tax provision in the ACA was the high-cost plan excise tax or the Cadillac tax, which will be discussed later in this chapter. It alone is projected to raise $111 billion from 2018 when it goes into effect through 2022 (Congressional Budget Office, 2012). ACA opponents have charged that these taxes on high-income earners and investment income will hinder economic growth; however, there is little indication this has been the case. Some analysts have also pointed out that contrary to Republican claims, the tax on so-called Cadillac insurance would not impact middle-class Americans. "These taxes are not likely to hit very many people in the middle class, if anybody," asserted Bob Williams of the Tax Policy Center (Contorno, 2014).

Nonetheless, the taxes and fees in the law became highly politicized issues, with updated estimates from CBO and JCT of the ACA reenergizing repeal attempts. Then House Budget Committee chairman (and former 2012 Republican Vice-Presidential candidate) Paul Ryan (R-WI) issued a press release after new CBO and JCT estimates on the fiscal impacts of the law, stating:

> The Congressional Budget Office reported today that the Affordable Care Act imposes a $1 trillion tax increase and continues to raid Medicare by over $700 billion to fuel a new $1.7 trillion open-ended entitlement, while doing nothing to reduce the backbreaking health care costs for families and businesses. . . . This law was built with smoke and mirrors to hide the impact of the trillions of dollars of new entitlement spending. . . . The only tool the President has left to prevent this entitlement from blowing another hole in the budget is massive tax increases and a board of fifteen unelected bureaucrats who will cut Medicare in ways that lead to denied care for seniors. . . . This future of diminished care is not what Americans deserve. The CBO's update—like the Supreme Court decision—only underscores the fact that it is up to the American people to repeal this misguided law and advance real health care reform. (Ryan, 2012)

The ACA includes a number of taxes and fees that affect nearly all sectors of the health care industry, as well as individuals. In particular, individuals earning more than $200,000 per year and families earning more than $250,000 are especially affected by new Medicare HI taxes. While the new taxes have proven to be as controversial as expected, they were critical to enacting a law that CBO and JCT projected would reduce the deficit.

FURTHER READING

Americans for Tax Reform. 2012. "Comprehensive List of Obama Tax Increases." Accessed April 14, 2015. http://s3.amazonaws.com/atrfiles/files/files/092712pr--Comprehensive%20Obama%20Tax%20Hike%20List.pdf.

Book, R. 2014. "How the ACA's Taxes Increase Premiums." American Action Forum. Accessed April 14, 2015. http://americanactionforum.org/research/how-the-acas-taxes-increase-premiums.

Burton, D. 2013. "Obamacare's Health Insurance Tax Targets Consumers and Small Businesses." The Heritage Foundation. Accessed April 14, 2015. http://www.heritage.org/research/reports/2013/10/obamacare-s-health-insurance-tax-targets-consumers-and-small-businesses.

Committee on Ways and Means. 2012. "CBO/JCT Confirm That Obamacare Is a $1 Trillion Tax Hike." Accessed April 14, 2015. http://waysand-means.house.gov/news/documentsingle.aspx?DocumentID=304547.

Congressional Budget Office. 2012. "Letter to the Honorable John Boehner." Accessed October 9, 2015. https://www.cbo.gov/sites/default/files/cbofiles/attachments/43471-hr6079.pdf.

Contorno, S. 2014. "Mitch McConnell Claims 'Devastating' Tax Increase on Middle Class Looming Due to Health Care Law." Politfact.com. Accessed July 10, 2015. http://www.politifact.com/truth-o-meter/statements/2014/jul/23/mitch-mcconnell/mitch-mcconnell-claims-devastating-tax-increase-mi/.

Hemmings, B., Fangmeier, J., and Udow-Phillips, M. 2013. "The Impact of ACA Taxes and Fees." Center for Health Care Research and Transformation. University of Michigan. Accessed April 14, 2015. http://www.chrt.org/publication/impact-aca-taxes-fees/.

The Heritage Foundation. 2012. "18 New Taxes and Penalties Totaling $836 Billion." Accessed April 14, 2015. http://thf_media.s3.amazonaws.com/2012/jpg/Obamacare%20in%20Pictures/special-obamacare-in-pictures-201210-08-HIRES.jpg.

Joint Committee on Taxation. 2010. "Estimated Revenue Effects of the Amendment in the Nature of a Substitute to H.R. 4872, The 'Reconciliation Act of 2010,' as Amended, in Combination with the Revenue Effects of H.R. 3590, the 'Patient Protection and Affordable Care Act' ('PPACA'), as Passed by the Senate and Scheduled for Consideration by the House Committee on Rules on March 20, 2010." Accessed April 14, 2014. https://www.jct.gov/publications.html?func=startdown&id=3672.

Ryan, P. 2012. "President's Health Care Law Remains a Fiscal Train Wreck." Accessed April 14, 2015. http://paulryan.house.gov/news/documentsingle.aspx?DocumentID=304468#.VS3C3fnF-g4.

S.Con.Res.13. 2009. "An Original Concurrent Resolution Setting Forth the Congressional Budget for the United States Government for Fiscal Year 2010, Revising the Appropriate Budgetary Levels for Fiscal Year 2009, and Setting Forth the Appropriate Budgetary Levels for Fiscal Years 2011 through 2014." Senate Budget Committee. Accessed April 14, 2015. https://www.congress.gov/bill/111th-congress/senate-concurrent-resolution/13/text#toc-IDD55C3062DBDA4891A4469F77AADCD7FC.

Q40. DOES THE AFFORDABLE CARE ACT REQUIRE ALL UNINSURED INDIVIDUALS TO BUY INSURANCE OR PAY A FINANCIAL PENALTY?

Answer: Yes, in most cases. Perhaps the single most controversial provision in the ACA has been the individual mandate, which requires all Americans (with exceptions) to have a basic level of health insurance coverage or pay a tax-based penalty. The individual mandate proved to be so controversial that a legal challenge to the provision made it to the Supreme Court in June 2012. While the Supreme Court upheld the constitutionality of the individual mandate, it has continued to be a contentious issue.

The purpose of the individual mandate was to incent individuals to purchase coverage in the health insurance exchanges—instead of waiting until they became sick to do so—or face a penalty. The concept of an individual mandate in the United States had its origins among conservative economists and policy experts in the late 1980s and 1990s, and the concept enjoyed significant Congressional Republican support during the Clinton health reform debate (Rovner, 2010; S.1730, 1993). However, conservative support for the mandate disappeared when it became part of the proposed health care reform package developed by the Obama Administration and Democrats on Capitol Hill. Republican opposition to the mandate has continued well past the Supreme Court ruling. On several occasions, in fact, Republicans have introduced legislation to repeal the mandate, even though it is critical to maintaining affordable premiums in the ACA's health insurance exchanges.

The Facts: The individual mandate went into effect in 2014 at the same time that the insurance market reforms and the coverage expansion went into effect. The mandate requires that all Americans purchase a basic level of health insurance coverage—or minimum essential coverage—or face a tax-based penalty that increases from 2014 through 2016. The policy reasons for including the individual mandate in health reform were clear. Insurance market reforms, such as prohibiting preexisting condition exclusions, would inevitably attract sicker individuals with health needs to purchase coverage through the exchanges. However, to maintain affordable premium prices, healthy individuals have to join the new exchange insurance risk pools as well. In the absence of an individual mandate, insurers could be faced with adverse selection in which individuals with health needs are more likely to purchase coverage than healthier individuals—resulting in higher premiums that could prove unsustainable over the long term and ultimately do lasting damage to the health care system.

However, there are exemptions from the mandate and penalty, including religious conscience, membership in a health care sharing ministry, membership in a federally recognized Indian tribe, income below the minimum threshold for filing a tax return, unaffordable coverage options, undocumented status, and a broad "hardship" exemption among others (Internal Revenue Service, 2015). CBO estimated that 30 million individuals will remain uninsured in 2016 and that the majority—or 87 percent—will quality for an exemption from the individual mandate penalty (Congressional Budget Office, 2014). As a result, a minority of the uninsured will actually pay a penalty for not having insurance coverage.

The controversy surrounding the individual mandate culminated in a Supreme Court hearing in March 2012—just two years after the law's

Table 8.1 ACA Individual Mandate Penalty Structure

Years	Penalty Level
2014	Higher of: • $95 per person, with a maximum penalty of $285, or • 1% of yearly household income, with a maximum penalty equal to the national average premium for a bronze plan
2015	Higher of: • $325 per person, with a maximum penalty of $975, or • 2% of yearly household income, with a maximum penalty equal to the national average premium for a bronze plan
2016	Higher of: • $695 per person (adjusted for inflation in subsequent years), or • 2.5% of yearly household income, with a maximum penalty equal to the national average premium for a bronze plan

Source: Public Law 111-148. (2010) The Patient Protection and Affordable Care Act.

passage. In the *National Federation of Independent Businesses v. Sebelius,* plaintiffs challenged the constitutionality of the individual mandate, as well as the Medicaid expansion. The lawsuits against both provisions began as soon as the law was passed, with the state of Florida filing a lawsuit against both provisions the very day the ACA was signed into law (Henry J. Kaiser Family Foundation, 2012). Florida's lawsuit eventually had 25 other states join; in addition, the National Federation of Independent Businesses filed a lawsuit against the mandate. The Supreme Court considered the cases together (Henry J. Kaiser Family Foundation, 2012).

In June 2012, the Supreme Court upheld the constitutionality of the individual mandate but struck down the requirement that all states must expand their Medicaid programs (or risk losing funding for their existing Medicaid programs). The 5–4 majority ruling upheld the individual mandate referencing Congress's power to levy taxes. The swift opposition and speed with which the cases went to the Supreme Court underscore the divisiveness over the individual mandate.

The political history of the individual mandate, however, is more complicated. The idea in the United States had its origins in the late 1980s and 1990s when a group of conservative economists and health policy experts came together to try to design a market-oriented, universal health care system (Rovner, 2010). One of those economists, Dr. Mark Pauly wrote a paper describing the individual mandate as an alternative to the employer mandates proposed by President Clinton (Pauly, 1994). In an interview after the ACA passed on the origins of the mandate, he stated that the reason for it was that "there would always be some Evel Knievels of health insurance, who would decline coverage even if the subsidies were very generous, and even if they could afford it, quote unquote, so if you really wanted to close the gap, that's the step you'd have to take" (Rovner, 2010). The individual mandate is regarded as a mechanism for increasing personal responsibility—so that individuals do not wait to purchase insurance until they need it. Support for the individual mandate extended beyond economists and policy experts, however. In 1993 Sen. Lincoln Chaffee (R-RI) sponsored the "Health Equity and Access Reform Today Act of 1993" (S.1730, 1993)—a Republican alternative to the Clinton health reform plan that included an individual mandate:

> The Secretary shall specifically make recommendations under paragraph (1) regarding establishing a requirement that all eligible individuals obtain health coverage through enrollment with a qualified health plan. (S.1730, 1993)

At the time, the legislation was cosponsored by prominent Republicans, including Senators Orrin Hatch (R-UT) and Charles Grassley (R-IA). In 2009–2010 both of these men were still in the Senate, and they both sat on that body's powerful finance committee. But their opposition to the ACA led them to denounce the very individual mandate that they had once praised. In 2009, days before the ACA passed the Senate, Sen. Orrin Hatch (R-UT) voiced his opposition to the individual mandate, "Congress has never crossed the line between regulating what people choose to do and ordering them to do it. The difference between regulating and requiring it is liberty" (Hatch, 2009).

In the years following the Supreme Court hearing, attempts to repeal the individual mandate have continued. In 2015, for example, Hatch and 27 Republican cosponsors introduced the "American Liberty Restoration Act," which would strike down the mandate. The Republican budget for 2016 also allows for the use of special legislative procedures with the stated intent of using them to repeal the ACA and the individual mandate.

If Republicans ever do succeed in ending the individual mandate, the impacts will be considerable. In 2012, CBO projected that eliminating the individual mandate would cause premiums in the individual health insurance exchanges to be 15 to 20 percent higher, given that younger and healthier individuals would forego coverage while less healthy individuals would retain their coverage (Banthin, 2012). CBO projected that this would reduce federal spending by $282 billion from 2012 to 2021 due to 12 million fewer individuals in exchange plans and Medicaid, and 4 million fewer individuals in employer-sponsored insurance—for a total of 16 million fewer individuals insured relative to current law (Banthin, 2012).

FURTHER READING

Banthin, J. 2012. "Effects of Eliminating the Individual Mandate to Obtain Health Insurance." Congressional Budget Office. Presentation at RAND BGOV Event on the Individual Mandate, March 20, 2012. Accessed April 15, 2015. http://cbo.gov/sites/default/files/cbofiles/attachments/RAND_BGOV_EliminatingIndividualMandate03-20.pdf.

Congressional Budget Office. 2014. "Payments of Penalties for Being Uninsured under the Affordable Care Act: 2014 Update." Accessed April 14, 2015. http://www.cbo.gov/sites/default/files/45397-IndividualMandate.pdf.

Hatch, O. 2009. Congressional Record-Senate, Vol. 155, Pr. 24. December 22, 2009.

Internal Revenue Service. 2015. "Questions and Answers on the Individual Shared Responsibility Provision." Accessed April 14, 2015. http://www.irs.gov/Affordable-Care-Act/Individuals-and-Families/Questions-and-Answers-on-the-Individual-Shared-Responsibility-Provision.

Henry J. Kaiser Family Foundation. 2012. "A Guide to the Supreme Court's Affordable Care Act Decision." Accessed April 15, 2015. https://kaiserfamilyfoundation.files.wordpress.com/2013/01/8332.pdf.

Pauly, M. 1994. "Making a Case for Employer-Enforced Individual Mandates." *Health Affairs*, Spring (II): 22–33. Accessed April 15, 2015. http://content.healthaffairs.org/content/13/2/21.full.pdf.

Public Law 111–148. (2010) The Patient Protection and Affordable Care Act.

Rovner, J. 2010. "Republicans Spurn Once-Favored Health Mandate." NPR. Accessed April 15, 2015. http://www.npr.org/templates/story/story.php?storyId=123670612.

S.40. 2013. "American Liberty Restoration Act." Accessed May 26, 2015. https://www.congress.gov/bill/113th-congress/senate-bill/40/text.

S.1730. 1993. "Health Equity and Access Reform Today Act of 1993." Accessed April 14, 2015. http://www.gpo.gov/fdsys/pkg/BILLS-103s1770pcs/pdf/BILLS-103s1770pcs.pdf.

Q41. WHAT IS THE SO-CALLED CADILLAC TAX CONTAINED IN THE AFFORDABLE CARE ACT?

Answer: One of the key long-term financing mechanisms in the ACA is an excise tax on high-cost plans—commonly referred to as the "Cadillac tax"—set to take effect in 2018. The excise tax targets so-called Cadillac plans, many of which offer generous health insurance benefits, with little to no cost-sharing to individuals. Economists theorize that these plans result in overutilization of services because individuals are not sensitive to the price of medical services, such as unnecessary tests and provider visits, which contribute to rising health care costs. While the term implies that a limited number of plans will be affected, surveys suggest that up to half of all employers will be affected by the Cadillac tax when it goes into effect in 2018 and over 80 percent could be affected by 2023 (Towers Watson, 2014). However, this assumes that employers will not make changes to benefits to avoid the tax, which most employers will do.

The Cadillac tax has been politically unpopular on both sides of the aisle—because it taxes employer-sponsored health benefits; however, the idea has had long-standing support among health economists as a mechanism for curbing overutilization of health services and making health care consumers more price sensitive. Attempts to delay or repeal the Cadillac tax are expected to intensify in the coming years as more employer plans are projected to be affected—especially union plans. However, the provision is critical to the ACA's potential for controlling long-term health care cost growth—as evidenced by CBO projecting it will save $149 billion starting when the tax goes into effect in 2018 to 2025 alone (Congressional Budget Office, 2015). Despite the political difficulties surrounding the provision, its potential to help control or constrain health care cost growth is at least one reason the Cadillac tax has not been amended.

The Facts: A series of tax and other policy decisions dating back to the 1930s gave rise to the system in the United States today in which approximately 50 percent—or 149 million Americans—receive coverage through employer-sponsored insurance (Henry J. Kaiser Family Foundation and Health Research and Educational Trust, 2014). The most critical policy decision was to make employer-sponsored health insurance benefits tax exempt in which the value of health insurance benefits is not counted as taxable income—a tax policy that eventually was estimated to cost the federal government $250 billion annually (Piotrowski, 2013). Economists have cited a number of problems with the tax-exempt status of employer-sponsored health insurance. First, the tax exemption disproportionately benefits those with higher incomes because they are subject to higher tax rates—and therefore receive the greatest benefit from untaxed compensation or benefits. On the other hand, those without employer-sponsored insurance receive no comparable tax benefit. Second—and perhaps more critically for the ACA—economists contend that the federal tax incentives encourage generous employer-sponsored health plans, which in turn drive up health care costs because they often cover a wide range of services, with minimal to no cost-sharing; as a result, individuals are not sensitive to the costs of the services they consume, leading to overutilization.

In an effort to bend the cost curve over the long term—and raise revenue to pay for the coverage expansion—Senate lawmakers opted to limit the open-ended tax exemption for employer-sponsored insurance. In the end, the provision was structured as an excise tax on high-cost plans. Specifically, the ACA imposes a 40 percent excise tax starting in 2018 on the cost of a health insurance plan that exceeds $10,200 for individual or $27,500 for family coverage. Each year the thresholds set in the ACA would be adjusted. In 2018 and 2019, the thresholds are indexed to the Consumer Price Index (CPI) plus 1 percent, and starting 2020 the thresholds are indexed to CPI alone. Both indices are below medical cost growth—and this was done deliberately to ensure the reduced deficit, and also to place increasing pressure on employer-sponsored insurance to slow premium growth and health care costs (Piotrowski, 2013). In 2012, two years after the ACA's passage, the JCT estimated that the Cadillac tax would raise $149 billion in revenues from 2018 to 2025, although this is still a fraction of what the overall tax-exempt status of employer-sponsored insurance costs the nation in terms of lost revenue (Joint Committee on Taxation, 2012). Interestingly, most of the revenue from this new tax comes from increased taxable income for individuals than from the excise tax itself.

However, in the winter of 2010 when Senate and House Democrats were negotiating each chamber's health reform legislation, the Cadillac tax became a serious point of contention. One of the key Democratic constituencies concerned about the provision was labor unions, as many members of those groups were projected to have plans that would be affected by the Cadillac tax. As a result, the Administration and Congressional Democrats agreed to modify the original Cadillac tax in the Senate legislation by increasing the thresholds and making adjustments for plans that are high cost not due to the generosity of benefits, but because they cover older, sicker individuals as well as policies that cover individuals in high-risk professions (e.g., firefighters, police officers).

Conservative health care experts have also alleged that because of the structure of the excise tax it would actually negatively impact lower-income individuals who receive more benefits in the form of a generous health insurance plan, rather than additional income (Capretta and Levin, 2014). However, a Republican alternative to the ACA, the Patient CARE Act, also includes capping the generosity of employer-sponsored health insurance benefits. A summary of the legislation states,

> We recognize that employer-sponsored insurance is an important feature of our health care system that provides coverage to nearly 150 million Americans, so we scrap the job-killing employer mandate and preserve the employer deduction. However, the open-ended tax preference encourages higher costs and increased spending. Our proposal maintains the employer deduction, so employers continue to have incentive to provide quality coverage to their employees. At the same time, we institute a cap on the exclusion for employees' health coverage valued at a generous $12,000 for an individual and $30,000 for a family and index it at CPI+1 for perpetuity. Unlike the punitive Cadillac Plan Tax in current law which imposes an

onerous excise tax of 40 percent on cost of coverage of health plans that exceed the annual limit, our proposal treats every additional dollar after the generous threshold at the individual's tax rate—a more balanced approach for middle class Americans. (Senate Finance Committee, 2015)

While the excise tax may not be the most effective structure for limiting the generosity of employer-sponsored benefits, Republican health reform and financing ideas are proposing to cap the exclusion as well.

As 2018 approaches, there is growing concern about how many employee plans could be subject to the excise tax—and many employers are restructuring benefits well in advance of 2018 to avoid the tax. A 2014 Towers Watson Survey found that nearly 75 percent of surveyed companies said they were very or somewhat concerned that they would trigger the tax and over 60 percent report that they believe it will have a moderate or great impact on their health care strategy in 2015 and 2016 (Towers Watson, 2014). The survey also reported that nearly 50 percent of respondents believe they were likely to trigger the tax in 2018 and 82 percent by 2023 (Towers Watson, 2014). The ACA's Cadillac tax does tax employer health benefits; however, the idea of limiting the open-ended tax treatment of employer sponsored insurance has been a bipartisan idea, with a long history of support from health economists due to its potential to recue health care cost growth into the future.

FURTHER READING

Capretta, J., and Levin, Y. 2014. "Getting There. Ethics and Public Policy Center." Accessed April 16, 2015. http://eppc.org/publications/getting-there/.

Congressional Budget Office, 2015. "The Budget and Economic Outlook: 2015 to 2025." Accessed April 16, 2015. https://www.cbo.gov/sites/default/files/cbofiles/attachments/49892-Outlook2015.pdf.

Henry J. Kaiser Family Foundation and Health Research Educational Trust. 2014. "Employer Health Benefits: 2014 Annual Survey." Accessed January 3, 2015. http://files.kff.org/attachment/2014-employer-health-benefits-survey-full-report.

Joint Committee on Taxation. 2012. "Revenue Estimates." June 15, 2012. Accessed April 14, 2015. http://waysandmeans.house.gov/uploadedfiles/jct_june_2012_partial_re-estimate_of_tax_provisions_in_aca.pdf.

Piotrowski, J. 2013. "Excise Tax on 'Cadillac' Plans. Health Policy Briefs." *Health Affairs*. Accessed April 16, 2015. http://www.healthaffairs.org/healthpolicybriefs/brief.php?brief_id=99.

Senate Finance Committee. 2015. "The Patient Choice, Affordability, Responsibility, and Empowerment Act." Accessed April 16, 2015. http://murphy.house.gov/uploads/TWO%20PAGER.pdf.

Towers Watson. 2014. "Nearly Half of U.S. Employers Expected to Hit the Health Care 'Cadillac' Tax in 2018 with 82% Triggering the Tax by 2023." Accessed April 15, 2015. http://www.towerswatson.com/en-US/Press/2014/09/nearly-half-us-employers-to-hit-health-care-cadillac-tax-in-2018-with-82-percent-by-2023.

Index

About the Author

Purva H. Rawal, PhD, has over a decade of health policy experience in academic, government, and private-sector settings. From 2005 to 2010, she served as staff in the U.S. Senate where she worked on the Senate Budget Committee as a key advisor to Chairman Kent Conrad (D-ND) during the drafting and passage of the Affordable Care Act. Prior to that, she was the health advisor to Sen. Joseph Lieberman (I-CT). After leaving Capitol Hill, Purva was Director at Avalere Health working on health reform implementation with health care industry and advocacy organizations.

She is currently a Principal at Capview Strategies, a health policy consultancy where she works with think tanks, health care coalitions, providers, payers and life sciences companies on health system payment and delivery reform and transformation issues. She is also an Adjunct Assistant Professor at Georgetown University, where she teaches undergraduate classes, including Politics of Health Care. She started her health policy career as a Christine Mirzayan Science and Technology Fellow at the National Academy of Sciences/National Academy of Medicine, and began on Capitol Hill as a Congressional Fellow for the Society for Research on Child Development and the American Association for the Advancement of Science.

Dr. Rawal holds a BA and PhD from Northwestern University and lives in Washington, DC, with her husband and two children.